Unraveled

Unraveled:

*Prescriptions to repair a
broken health care system*

Dr. William B. Weeks and Dr. James N. Weinstein

This book is dedicated to Shelsey Weinstein, Brieanna's sister.
Tikkun Olam.
~JNW

This book is dedicated to Hoke and Joplin.
Thanks for being there.
~WBW

Contents

Notes from the Authors

A Personal Narrative for Real Change

I have had a very personal—and unfortunate—health care experience, one that has transformed my life and that of my family forever, and has encouraged me to write this book. I want others to better grasp the challenges inherent in the current health care system, to see what is possible, and to understand why health care delivery needs to move from a system based on volume to a system of value based on outcomes. We need a sustainable system that is focused on improving the health of communities and populations and not on growing market share; a system that moves away from fee-for-service reimbursement—where doing more, regardless of outcomes, results in higher incomes—toward reimbursement contingent on achieving the best possible outcomes at the lowest possible cost.

Our daughter Brieanna, was an incredibly beautiful child, inside and out; she was a child with sparkling blue eyes, curly hair, and a smile that would light up any room she would enter. She was the light of my life and that of my incredible wife, Mimi. Like all parents of a firstborn, our dreams and hopes were bundled in this package of pure joy…She was simply perfect. She was our future; we began planning for her future the day she was born, and we envisioned that her future would be even better than ours. My brother and I were the first in our family to graduate from college, and we both became doctors. My wife and I saw Brieanna as capable of becoming anything she wanted, and we imagined she would be a great neurosurgeon. Admittedly, dreaming big is what all parents do with their children. But then one sunny day in spring of 1984, when Brieanna was 13 months old, she was diagnosed with leukemia: cancer, every parent's worst nightmare. What were we to do? I told Mimi, "We're at a great academic medical center, with the very best doctors; we can fix this, and she'll be OK…won't she?"

Over the next 12 years, Mimi and I would experience health care, and the system in which I have chosen to work for decades, from a very different perspective than any we'd had before Brieanna's illness. Seeing this system through the eyes of a parent of a very vulnerable child opened my eyes to so much that I had never seen as a health care provider. As a spine surgeon, my practice focused on patients with cancer of the spine. I had developed the worldwide classification for treating spine tumors, and certainly, I understood what was possible in cancer treatment. I figured that I, as well as anyone, would understand what patients and families were experiencing. However, as the treatments began, we realized how much health care—including health care decisions—would be out of our control. From the first day of her diagnosis, our belief in God was challenged in ways we couldn't have imagined. As time went by, days became weeks, weeks became months, and months became years of fear and lack of control, with a growing realization that, despite our best efforts and total compliance with the treatments offered, Brieanna might not survive. Mimi and I saw our beautiful bundle of joy get increasingly sick, not just from this terrible disease, but from the intense chemotherapeutic and radiation treatments she had to endure virtually every day: treatments that are both difficult to understand and pronounce and that had an intensity that would challenge any mortal, let alone a young child. Brieanna lost her beautiful auburn hair; she got sores in her mouth and could not eat; she had to spend several days a month in a hospital; she became susceptible to life-threatening infections because the treatments compromised her immune system. So we had to restrict her activities. The joy of a visit from a family member or a friend was greatly dampened by a deep concern that the visit might make her sick and land her back in the hospital.

We religiously followed the prescribed course of treatment for nearly 12 long years. At each anniversary of her diagnosis, Mimi and I prayed that this would be the year when Brie would get better, could play carefree, could enjoy life like her friends did, and could get back to becoming that neurosurgeon we knew she would be. Brie did well for various periods over these years. But the cancer came back five different times, and each time, the doctors told us we needed to start over. Each time our spirits were tested beyond what seemed possible, and each time we wondered how much more Brie could take. The treatments were robbing Brie of the most simple joys, and they were getting more intense; brain and spine radiation was added with each relapse that involved cancer within the central nervous system. We wondered how God could do this to an innocent child, who never hurt anyone, and who hadn't even had a chance to live a normal life.

From my professional training, I knew that brain and spine radiation in a child could have devastating long-term consequences because the nerve cells are still growing and forming connections. An additional problem is that radiation can induce new, different tumors—so the treatments can themselves worsen the disease. Mimi and I wondered whether alternative therapies might be considered.

But any hesitation in continuing the prescribed course of treatment was met with incredible resistance and even threats of lawsuits. We were told that if we would not agree to recommended treatments, then we were not allowing the best things for our daughter. In this horrible period of our lives, the very doctors whom we respected as colleagues and friends told us that they would sue us if we did not comply with their recommendations for continued radiation and complicated protocols; yet they could offer no guarantees.

Brie died a few months before her 12th birthday. As a dad, I fear I did not provide the best advice and decisions for my wife and daughter in an all-too-complicated health care system that seemed intent on providing treatments that we all knew could be futile, that might briefly extend life, but would have devastating side effects that would be too excessive for Brie and our family to endure. My wife and I, and her beloved little sister Shelsey, loved every minute we had with Brie, and we only wish we had had more time with her, a wish experienced by all families who lose a child. We love her and miss her and wish for others in our situation a calmness and easier path.

And that is why I wanted to write this book. This experience forever changed the lens through which I see the health care system. I became aware of a tremendous shortfall in American medicine. While we have incredible technology and have made major strides in applying that technology, providing high-quality care is so much more than applying technological interventions. Providing high-quality care involves understanding the whole patient: his or her values, environment, wants, and needs. That part of Brie's treatment was missing.

And this perspective has also been molded by my research experiences, wherein I have studied the tremendous unwarranted variations in the processes, costs, and outcomes of health care delivery provided across the United States. I have tried to address these issues by developing the first-in-the-nation "Center for Shared Decision Making"—a center that works to understand patient values, needs, and desires before recommending treatment—within the Dartmouth-Hitchcock Health System. In the 1980s, I developed and promoted the use of Patient-Reported Outcomes, and I have been able to leverage information technology to use these to help patients anticipate the outcomes of different treatment choices and thereby make informed health care decisions. As a leader of the High Value Healthcare Collaborative, I have worked to collaboratively improve health care outcomes and reduce health care costs in markets that serve one-fifth of the U.S. population. As the CEO and president of the Dartmouth-Hitchcock Health System, I am working to develop health care delivery and reimbursement models that no longer interfere with what should be the central focus of health care delivery—the relationship between a provider and a patient. And, as a physician who continues to see patients, I try in every interaction to give my patients the kind of health care experience they deserve, with them at the center of their care.

It is my hope that this book will help readers identify the current problems in health care delivery, will provide some understanding of how those problems came to be and the forces that keep them in place, and most importantly, will provide solutions to improve the existing system now, today, as we move to a much-needed revolution in health and health care delivery.

There is a better way. My family's experience with health care should not be the norm. I hope this book helps transform the normative experience to one that I know will be refreshing, supportive, engaged, efficient, and effective.

Dr. James N. Weinstein

 CEO and President, Dartmouth-Hitchcock Health System
 Past Director of the Dartmouth Institute for Health Policy and Clinical Research
 Peggy Y. Thomson Professor, the Geisel School of Medicine at Dartmouth
 Member, National Academy of Medicine

A Vision for the Future

I am thrilled to have this opportunity to write a book with Jim—I have been a longtime admirer of his vision, his passion, and his work. As a researcher Jim has inspired me to study better ways to deliver health care; as a leader, he has helped me understand the need for—and the challenges inherent in—transparently reporting health care outcomes and costs; as a collaborator, he has helped me grasp how to use that information to drive efficient and effective patient-centered health care delivery.

I have been fortunate in that my children have not had horrific health care experiences. But I am deeply concerned about the legacy that the health care system will leave their generation, if it continues operating as it has. Despite a recent slowdown in health care expenditures, the United States continues to spend an inordinate amount of its scarce resources on health care. As a proportion of our gross national product, we spend about twice what the next highest spending country does on health care.

And our outcomes are worse.

We have higher rates of childhood death. We have shorter lifespans. We have more obesity and heart disease and diabetes. And while we have the technology and capacity to address each of these life-taking disorders effectively, our health care system is not organized in a way that allows it to do so.

The irony is that America has the best health care available in the world—it has pockets of excellence wherein exceptionally well-delivered high-value care is the norm. But it also has enormous problems with access to care, the ability to consistently delivery high-value care, and waste. Health care systems that provide high-value health care are paid the same as those that do not; providers with abysmal outcomes continue to practice; and higher expenditures are associated with worse health outcomes, not better ones.

I fear that if we do not get health care costs under control—now—the debt that will continue to be created will bankrupt the next generation, a generation already hampered by very high levels of school debt. Further, because of the ineffectiveness of health care spending, the same kinds of health problems that challenge us today will only increase in the future, thereby exacerbating the fiscal problems.

Our inefficient and yet potentially tremendously effective health care system represents an opportunity. If we focus on learning from high-value health care systems to adopt what works and jettison what does not, our health care costs will shrink as the health of the nation improves; we will have a healthier workforce that can compete more effectively in the international marketplace, with products that are not overpriced because of embedded health care costs. America will continue to be a rich and productive country. But if we do not take this opportunity to rein in health care spending and invest more wisely in promoting the health of the population, the future success of our economy is jeopardized.

As we show in this book, we have the tools necessary to improve health care efficiency. We know what works, and just as importantly, we know what does not. We need to install required supportive structures, carefully evaluate the effectiveness of health interventions, deploy what works, show the results of that deployment, and work together to improve the nation's health.

I hope this book provides some guidance on how, exactly, to do that.

William B. Weeks, MD, PhD, MBA

Senior Researcher, the Dartmouth Institute for Health Policy and Clinical Practice

Professor, the Geisel School of Medicine at Dartmouth

2015–16 Tocqueville-Fulbright Distinguished Chair,
Aix-Marseille University, Marseille, France

Introduction

We have a major problem in the United States, and we are all aware of it. We spend far too much money on health care, and the impact of all that spending varies significantly based on where one lives and where one obtains care. Few players in the health care arena — whether patients, providers, or payers — are satisfied; most find the current construct of health care delivery inconvenient, incoherent, and even scary. Patients often feel ignored and treated like a number. Much like their assessment of their own congressional representatives and Congress, they seem to like their own doctor, but they understand that the system is broken. They have had — or they have friends who have had — upsetting encounters with the health care system: encounters where their records were unavailable, making them concerned that they might not be getting the right care; encounters where they were overdiagnosed, misdiagnosed, or got inappropriate or too much treatment; and encounters (almost all of them) where they receive an incomprehensible bill.

Like the Rosetta Stone when first discovered, much of medicine appears to be indecipherable; care delivery is far too complex, and it is difficult to know what care one should receive, what care one should avoid, and who is in charge of the care provided. And while health care reform has increased the number of people with health insurance coverage, it has added to this complexity, creating yet another layer of language and structure that few can understand — language and structure that might be impermeable to more vulnerable populations — thereby creating a wider gap between those with and without health care literacy. Many patients have pursued and adhered to treatment plans only to later discover better alternatives to the care plan they had been offered. They had simply not been offered those alternatives, and they never understood the true risks, benefits, potential outcomes, or out-of-pocket costs for the care they were provided. Many patients have experienced adverse events, unnecessary admissions, and medication errors. They have seen the impact of unwarranted and expensive end-of-life care and they have seen chronic-care problems mismanaged. Most patients have no "trusted navigator" to help with their health care decision-making.

Providers are not happy, either. They are distracted by more and more administrative work; they do not feel supported by the health care system in which they work; and they know the system can be better. The vast majority of health care providers pursued their professions to help people. But physicians find that the current administrative structures, regulations, and health care delivery processes interfere with their ability to help those most in need. Further, they see the financial rewards of their work accrue to drug manufacturers, insurers, and device companies. In the last decade, the costs of attending medical school have vastly outstripped growth in primary care physician salaries; meanwhile, the salaries of CEOs of insurance agencies, pharmaceutical manufacturers, and health care delivery systems have skyrocketed. It continues to be difficult to persuade medical or advanced nursing students to enter primary care fields because the hours are overwhelming, primary care physicians' satisfaction levels are low, and when compared to specialist physicians' income, their incomes are low.

The inability to attract medical and advanced nursing students into primary care fields is worrisome because the success of the Affordable Care Act (ACA) is premised on having ready access to primary care providers. However, the ACA does not discourage overuse of care, poor coordination of care, or use of ineffective care. So, although the ACA has increased insurance coverage and access through subsidies and exchanges, the United States will continue to spend more than 17 percent of its gross domestic product on health care—by far, the highest in the industrialized world. Further, by continuing to shift costs of care to patients (by increasing insurance copayments and deductibles), health care consumers will experience higher out-of-pocket health care costs going forward. In addition, states will not be able to afford their ever-increasing Medicaid budgets, which will mean that individuals' tax burdens will increase or Medicaid benefits will become diminished.

We are facing a dire national crisis.

Patients and providers might ask, "How did we get here? And what's the alternative?"

As it turns out, there are a lot of reasons why health care has evolved to become the way it is. Just as Darwin found that animals in the Galapagos Islands adapted to their environments in different ways, health care has evolved in response to political and environmental changes and will likely continue to do so. This adaptation has not necessarily been in the best interests of patients. We think it is important to underscore these factors because changes in the models of care delivery that they have produced will be required for the health care system to adapt in order to more effectively and efficiently deliver health care services in the future. In this book, we hope to paint a picture of the possible, where new models that promote patients' best interests are merged with the best of advanced consumer-based technology to deliver care and improve health.

To paint this picture in this book, we use vignettes to identify problems inherent in the health care delivery services industry, explain why and how it got to be as it is, and offer practical, immediately applicable solutions designed to address these problems while reducing overall health care costs.

There is a better way, and we invite you to consider these solutions to imagine what the future of health care delivery might be. Just as the industrial revolution of the late 1700s—with new technologies and new methods of organizing the workforce—dramatically enhanced production and transformed how people worked, lived, and consumed products, a revolution in the way health care is produced, delivered, and consumed needs to happen. If done correctly, this revolution could lead America and the rest of the world toward a new system of health care that is built around improving the health of the population: a system that incorporates new technologies—drawn from within and outside of medicine—and leverages new partnerships to deliver health care in a more effective, efficient, and consumer-friendly fashion. The transformation of health care delivery will be tumultuous and many vested interests will resist the change. But change is possible. And it is critical to the creation of a sustainable health care system that is affordable, transparent, and effective at compassionately treating patients who are ill and keeping those people who are not ill, healthy.

Now is the time for change. If we do not foster this industrial revolution in health care, U.S. health care costs will continue to rise, we will impoverish our children, we will not be competitive in the world marketplace, and our patients will suffer. Successful transformation of the health care system will require collaboration with new, as well as established, players in the health care marketplace. We believe this industrial revolution in health care will help create healthy, happier societies, will restore joy and meaning to clinical work, and will produce much greater returns on health care investments.

We welcome you to join us on this exciting journey.

Chapter 1

Access

Sandy was a divorced mother of three who lived in rural New Hampshire. In high school she was doing well and planning to go to college, but she got pregnant and had her first child, a boy, with Dean. After a year together, Dean decided he could not handle the responsibility of parenting, so he moved to California. Receiving only $25 a week in child support, Sandy got a job at a convenience store, but the childcare cost her about one-third of her income. About a year after Dean left, Sandy married Joe, and they had two little girls. But Joe was a somewhat violent alcoholic. They separated, and he left for a job in Texas; he provided $150 per week in child support. Sandy moved in with her parents, and her mom helped her some with the childcare. Sandy had three part-time jobs, none of which provided employer-sponsored health insurance. Across these three jobs, she worked between 50 and 60 hours a week for an hourly wage. .If she took time off work, she lost income.

Sandy had access to health insurance through New Hampshire Medicaid. After discussion with a friend of hers who lived across the river in Vermont, Sandy found out that New Hampshire Medicaid insurance provided substantially fewer benefits to her and her children than Vermont Medicaid did. Although she had considered it in the past, Sandy could not move to Vermont right then for several reasons. First, she was worried that the fathers of her children would not be cooperative with the move (she would have to notify them and they would have to agree to the move). Second, living with her parents saved her a lot of money and she was not sure she could afford to move to Vermont. Finally, she would have to get new childcare and new jobs, and she was concerned she might not be able to find either in Vermont.

Sandy's mother was a breast cancer survivor, so Sandy knew she was at high risk and needed to get screened regularly for breast and cervical cancer. However, she had not seen a physician in about five years, since her last child was born. While her children had received all of their vaccinations for school, and she made sure to get them to the pediatrician once a year, Sandy had found it hard to find a primary care physician for herself. Her former doctor had been working in a rural setting as part of a loan repayment program and had relocated four years before. While a new provider had recently opened a practice a few towns away, that provider did not take Medicaid patients. A larger health care system that was about an hour and a half away had a low-cost, "high-risk" health program for women, but Sandy would have to miss almost a day of work to go there. Plus, she was not sure her car would survive the trip.

She decided to wait until the next year to try to schedule an appointment for herself to see if her financial situation improved.

During that year Sandy developed a lump in her breast, and by the time she could get in to see a primary care physician, her nipple was secreting blood. She was diagnosed with stage three adenocarcinoma of the breast. She received chemotherapy and radiation therapy, and she lost all her jobs. Two years later, she died of metastatic breast cancer after generating over $1 million in bills.

How We Got Here

While health insurance was not widely available or used before World War II, since then, health insurance in the United States has been linked to employment. During World War II, wage freezes led employers to offer health insurance in order to attract workers—who were in short supply, because of the war—into their employ. After World War II, health insurance became a fairly standard benefit among larger employers for full-time workers. Because U.S. productivity and the U.S. economy boomed after World War II, there were few concerns about the growth of this new benefit. Since this new method of insurance paid providers "usual and customary charges," physicians embraced it; previously, they might have rendered services and then not gotten paid for them.

However, concerns grew that retired employees, who no longer had access to employer-sponsored health insurance, might not have access to health care services. In 1965, as part of the Great Society initiative, Congress established two government programs that were designed to provide health care insurance to patients who were either aged 65 and older or disabled (Medicare) or who were poor (Medicaid). Medicare, which is a federally run program, is a retirement and disability benefit that is still contingent on employment; employees must pay a percentage of their income for 10 years in order to become eligible for the program. Sixty-five was chosen as the age of Medicare eligibility for two reasons: that was a traditional retirement age, and that was also about the average lifespan at the time. The idea was that people would pay into the program, but not everyone would live to take full advantage of it. And without the advanced, expensive, and life-sustaining technology that has been developed over the past 50 years, Medicare might have continued to be effectively and sustainably funded this way. Medicaid, too, was funded through taxes on wages, but the program was to be run by state governments, so that it could be most responsive to the needs of the local population. However, considerably different benefits and eligibility criteria were offered in different states, perhaps generating geographic-based disparities in access to care.

Physician groups vehemently opposed the establishment of these federal programs, fearful of government price setting. Until about 1981, with the establishment of diagnosis related groups (DRGs), price setting did not happen; reimbursement had been based on historical health care charges, and this resulted in rapid growth in health care expenditures. Despite efforts to curtail this cost growth, medical expenditures have accelerated at a rate that is much higher than inflation and have consumed more and more of the American gross domestic product. Fueled by expensive technology, lack of restraint in health services demand, and perhaps overuse of testing and procedures, this unsustainable growth has also occurred in both employer-sponsored health insurance groups and in Medicare. As can be seen in **Figure 1,** while inflation in per-capita Medicare expenditures far outpaces that for general inflation, life expectancy has only shown a modest increase.

Figure 1. Relative changes in per-capita Medicare expenditures, the consumer price index, and life expectancy at age 65, 1970–2010.

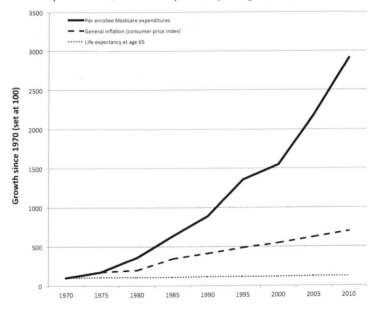

The most common mechanism of payment for health care services today continues to be fee-for-service, wherein physicians and providers are reimbursed based on specific services they provide. High-technology interventions are reimbursed at higher rates than preventive care. To date, providers have not been paid for the following: care coordination (e.g., ensuring that documents are sent to specialists or that follow-up care is rapidly provided following hospitalization), care that does not involve a face-to-face visit (such as telephone calls or e-mails), or the quality of care that is provided (such as whether they appropriately refer patients, follow evidence-based guidelines, or give vaccinations). Today it is much easier for consumers to know what is inside a cereal box (due to the required food labeling standards, enforced by the Food and Drug Administration) than it is for patients to know what his or her doctor's or health system's results are. Because different insurances pay different amounts for the same services, providers can preferentially provide care to those with good insurance. Historically, this has resulted in less access to care for those on Medicaid, which is generally one of the lowest reimbursing health insurances.

Preventive care consists of measures taken for disease prevention, while illness care consists of treatment for identified diseases or disorders. Preventive care includes recommended vaccines and laboratory or physical examination screening. Illness care might include diabetes management or heart surgery. It is sometimes difficult to get preventive care, particularly for those without good insurance, although the Affordable Care Act is improving access to such care. But emergent and illness care tends to be easier to access. Our health care system has been built around a hospital- and specialty-care nexus. Primary care and prevention, despite their cost effectiveness, can sometimes seem to be an afterthought, and therefore less important. Nothing could be further from the truth. And lack of easy access to primary care unfortunately makes Sandy's story a common one; before the financial crisis, the most common reason for declaring bankruptcy was because of health care bills, many of which might have been avoided had better access to primary care and preventive health care services been available.

What to Do

Before we can address challenges in the step-by-step process of health care delivery that we examine in the rest of the book, we have to address the challenge of being able to get into the health care system. Certainly, a number of federal and state programs exist to try to improve access to care for people like Sandy: Medicaid specifically targets the poor; Medicare eligibility is available for those who are determined to be disabled; Federally Qualified Health Centers provide subsidized care for the poor; and a number of federally funded programs—such as the Indian Health Service, the Veterans Health Administration, and the State Children's Health Insurance Program (SCHIP)—target individuals who have particular characteristics and who may be poor. But with each of these programs comes a bureaucratic burden that drives up health care costs and may represent barriers to access for the very patients these programs are to serve. There are forms to be completed, challenges in finding sites that will accept the type of insurance that the program provides, long distances in order to access care for some programs, and frequently, substantial waiting periods between the time of application and the time when a patient can access care. Just having some sort of health insurance coverage does not guarantee that providers will accept that insurance, and if they do, that they will provide high-quality health care. Good insurance does not necessarily equate to good health care.

Historically, patients who have restricted access to primary care have used emergency rooms to treat acute illnesses, but the expenditures for such care are phenomenally high and are largely considered wasteful for two reasons. First, most of these cases might have been treated equally well in a lower acuity setting, such as a doctor's office, had the patient been able to easily access primary care. Second, when the cases have become severe enough to warrant a visit to the emergency room, often an earlier intervention—or even preventive care—could have curtailed the progression of the malady.

So, to address the issues of access to health care that Sandy's case raises, patients need to have ready access to primary care providers—including physicians, nonphysician providers, and community health workers—and they need to have access to preventive testing and treatment that could thwart the progression of life-threatening diseases. These types of services should be free to all, so that patients do not experience personal financial hardship to get them. Further, these types of services should be adequately reimbursed so that more providers will accept patients who need their services and so that more providers will enter the primary care fields. Ideally, these services would be readily available at convenient locations and times—even in the workplace, if possible—so that patients do not face direct and indirect costs in getting the care that they need.

Perhaps one of the most effective ways of achieving these goals is to change the incentives that patients, providers, and employers now have. Currently, the predominant fee-for-service model incentivizes providers to provide more services, especially those that pay better. Since interventions for acute-care needs generally are reimbursed more than those for preventive care, these acute-care services "squeeze out" the availability of preventive care services; providers are more willing to provide the acute-care services. But if providers of all types were paid on a capitated basis—that is to say that providers would get a single payment for all the care that a patient receives over a specified time period—the providers would have an incentive to ensure that patients get the preventive care they need. This approach would have long-standing benefits for the nation, generating tremendous long-term payoffs by treating patients early and eliminating the need for more expensive care that is provided later to fix ills that might have been avoided in the first place. To further improve access to preventive care, those capitated payments might be modified based on how effective providers are at ensuring that their patients get recommended preventive care. Indeed, future reimbursement might be designed so that higher performance (publicly documented with easily interpretable measures, just as cereal boxes report nutritional information) would result in higher capitated reimbursement rates or supplements for excellent performance.

And employers, even those who have part-time workers, might have incentives for ensuring that their employees have access to free preventive care. One might imagine a reduced tax rate or lower health plan premiums for employers who provide access to such care. Alternatively, health plans might give employers a subsidy for providing on-site access to primary and preventive care at the workplace in order to encourage employees to use these services. These federal or commercial investments would pay off in the long run, as preventive care would decrease later demand for high-cost interventional care.

Finally, the mix of physicians who go into primary care versus specialty care is not ideal. Currently, students are entering specialty care at about five times the rate that they enter primary care. Yet, when an area has more primary care physicians, a number of studies have shown that overall costs of care are lower, health care outcomes are better, and unwarranted admissions to the hospital (which reflect a failure of outpatient care) are fewer.

A number of factors influences why physicians pick a particular specialty area. Primary care physicians are generally paid less, have a lower return on their educational investment, are less highly regarded, and report having less control over their life and work schedule than do specialty care physicians. These issues could be addressed if current payment schemes that seemingly overpay specialist physicians and underpay primary care physicians were to be rectified (currently, the average annual income of primary care physicians is about one-third that of specialty care physicians). Further, new models of health care delivery that support primary care physicians could help them maintain a sense of control over their lives and preserve their ability to derive joy from the practice of medicine.

Each of these solutions is possible, and a number have been tried. The biggest challenge seems to be to unseat the vested interests that strive to keep the current practices in place. Some non-primary care specialty groups have lobbyists that are among the most powerful in Washington, whose goal is to sustain high levels of reimbursement for interventions and procedures.

The Affordable Care Act has largely made health insurance more accessible and affordable for more people. However, its success is predicated on having an adequate supply of primary care providers. Further, patients like Sandy will likely continue to have difficulties justifying out-of-pocket expenditures for health procedures such as screening tests and physical exams. This is because, in response to increases in health insurance costs, many employers have adopted policies that transfer more out-of-pocket costs to their employees or have increased the number of part-time positions in their workforces, so that they are not required to provide access to health insurance, as they are for full-time workers.

More promising would be models of health care delivery and health promotion that are designed to serve a defined population and that put providers at risk for ensuring the care they pro-vide is effective and efficiently delivered. Then, if reimbursement were modified to encourage access to — and use of — preventive, non-hospital-based care, and if health care utilization, costs, and outcomes were transparently reported, consumers could make informed decisions about whether and where to obtain particular health care services. Further, the demand for primary care providers would grow, as would their status, so that more medical students, nursing graduates, and an evolving new health and health care workforce would enter primary care. To effectively support primary care providers, this new workforce would include a new breed of technical support staff and would leverage the use of sensor devices—wearable or usable devices that collect and can transmit health-relevant data—that would be securely connected to datasets. Then, embedded analytic capabilities would revolutionize health care delivery by working to prevent illness and maintain wellness instead of simply treating patients who present as sick or injured.

Over time, as preventive care interventions reduce the risk of acute-care episodes being needed in the community, expensive assets such as operating rooms, hospital beds, and intensive care units would be needed less. This would encourage continued growth of primary care and preventive services while decreasing per capita costs. Then, the revolution from a fee-for-service illness-based production model to a capitated health production model would be complete.

These kinds of changes would be accompanied by many new entrants into the health and health care markets: technological, biological, and phenotypic information datasets would be linked to a growing body of genomic, proteomics, and metabolic information to allow targeted immunological and viral treatments at the individual level. New businesses should stimulate the economy and generate less harmful, but more effective, diagnostic and treatment modalities, many of which will be available in patients' homes.

We believe it is time for a revolution in health and health care that is similar in scope and impact to the industrial revolution that transformed America in the late 1700s. We can no longer support the current arcane and ineffective health care system and suffer the financial losses fostered by the fee-for-service payment system.

And if we were able to execute this revolution, over time, preventable tragedies like Sandy's should disappear.

Chapter 2

Initial Encounter/ Waiting Room

John Henderson had been referred by his primary care provider, Dr. Jefferies, to an orthopedic surgeon for evaluation of chronic knee pain and possible knee replacement surgery. Dr. Jefferies said he had sent Dr. Lilly, the orthopedic surgeon, all the relevant records, including copies of two MRIs that John had gotten in the last couple of years. John had just had his annual physical exam, including blood tests, and everything but the knee was normal. For a 62-year-old man, John was in fabulous shape. The only reason he wanted to get evaluated for a knee replacement is because a series of analgesic trials and even joint injections had been unsuccessful in controlling his knee pain. The pain was increasingly impeding John's ability to stay active: he worked out daily, had recently retired, and planned to spend his retirement completing walking tours all over the world with his wife.

About two weeks before his appointment with Dr. Lilly, John received some forms in the mail asking about his health and knee pain. These were the same forms he'd just completed at his annual physical with Dr. Jefferies, but he completed them again. The instructions indicated that he should bring the completed forms to the appointment.

John arrived at Dr. Lilly's office 30 minutes early. He checked in with the receptionist and handed in his forms. The receptionist gave him another set of forms. "These are about your past medical history," she said.

"I think Dr. Jefferies sent over my records," John said.

"He did, but everyone has to fill out the forms."

As John was completing the forms, he noticed that several were similar to the ones that he'd just handed to the receptionist.

Some of the forms have changed," she said, when John asked whether there'd been a mistake.

About 45 minutes after his appointment was to have begun, John was brought into the exam room and given a gown. He wore shorts to the appointment, because he figured Dr. Lilly would want to examine his knee.

"Do I really need to put this on?" he asked.

"Yes," the receptionist said.

When Dr. Lilly came into the room, John was sitting on the exam table in the gown.

"Hello, John. I'm Dr. Lilly. What are we here for today?"

"I've had knee pain for some time—Dr. Jefferies referred me to you. He said that he'd sent over the records."

"I'm sure he did, but I like to hear things right from the patient's mouth. So, can you tell me a bit about your medical history?"

"I'm happy to, but I filled out several forms, and I think Dr. Jefferies provided a summary. I'm actually meeting my wife in about 30 minutes—I thought this would take less time."

Well, before we figure out what to do about your knee pain, we need to see whether you're healthy—whether you've got heart disease or hypertension or diabetes or anything. And we've got to figure out whether we should consider more conservative measures. Not everyone should get surgery."

John was a little frustrated. "So, over the past several years, my knee pain has gotten worse, as has my MRI. We've tried analgesics, steroid injections, and gel injections, but the pain continues. I'm in excellent health."

Well, let me look over the records and determine that," Dr. Lilly said.

After spending about 20 more minutes with Dr. Lilly, John had conveyed all the information that he'd provided on the forms and that he was sure would have been included in any summary Dr. Jefferies would have provided. John had to cancel his plans for lunch with his wife, as Dr. Lilly wanted to review the records that Dr. Jefferies had sent.

After waiting another 15 minutes, Dr. Lilly returned. "It looks like you're a pretty good historian — your summary was exactly consistent with what Dr. Jefferies described. But I'm a bit confused. The records indicate that you are a physician yourself — you recently retired after practicing internal medicine for 25 years...Why didn't you tell me you were a doctor?"

"You never asked," John said.

How We Got Here

Health care has long been focused around health care providers. Certainly, providers have worked long and hard hours, but in an effort to improve their efficiency, they began to centralize their practices in offices and hospitals instead of making house calls. From an efficiency standpoint, that made a lot of sense. As physicians became more specialized and medical equipment became more expensive, it became important to use these scarce resources efficiently. Over time it became impractical for physicians to spend time traveling to their patients (and then to be unavailable if an emergency arose), and it was impossible to move expensive equipment to patients.

Additionally, patient information has long been the sine qua non of medical practice. While novel technologies that were designed to improve diagnostic and therapeutic effectiveness have been developed, the foundation of good medical practice has always been to get an excellent history from the patient and to conduct a thorough physical exam — the "lost art" of medicine. Yet today, during the average patient visit, face-to-face contact with a doctor lasts only six minutes. A patient who lives in a rural setting might have to wake up at 4 a.m., drive several hours, find a parking space, spend 20 minutes finding the office in the hospital, and then have a six-minute interaction with the doctor. Sadly, this happens every day.

As health care expenditures have exploded over the past 60 years and government has assumed an ever-increasing role in health care payment, oversight, and regulation, there have been considerable advancements in medicine and technology around diagnosis and treatments that have saved lives and improved outcomes for critically ill patients; today, our military personnel are less likely to die in the field, car accidents are less likely to be fatal, and regularly we hear of cures for some cancers.

Yet these benefits are offset by setbacks. With the vast amount of information available, it is hard to keep up with technological advancements, and some organizations do not have the capital structures to do so. Indeed, there continues to be wide variation in the provision and outcomes of some services, potentially accelerated by this inability to keep abreast of new technologies and best practices. Further, more and more paperwork is required to maintain regulatory compliance, and more and more of the burden of completing that paperwork falls to patients. Patients like John are required to complete form after form—sometimes the same one—and yet the information is seemingly not used.

The information problem has been greatly accelerated as physicians continue to specialize and different payers require different information, forcing patients to go to multiple places to receive the full complement of health care services—imaging in radiology, blood tests at the laboratory, doctor visits in the clinic, preoperative scheduling at the hospital, and post-operative recovery in a skilled nursing facility. The challenge with so much information and with so many sites of care provision is that it is too overwhelming for providers who rely on just the most recent records. Transcription errors are made, and important factual information—such as the correct dose of a medication that a patient is taking or a list of medications to which a patient is allergic—sometimes might be buried in the chart. This has led to medical errors and in too many cases, harm to patients. Efforts to correct the root cause of the problem have included the implementation of electronic medical records and some protocols.

While the electronic medical record holds much promise, that promise has not yet been realized. To be sure, computer order entry by physicians has reduced transcription errors and errors in calculating dosing or in prescribing medications that are incompatible with one another. However, much of the electronic medical record is text-based, not numeric or quantifiable in usual ways, so incomprehensible volumes of unusable data are still included in a patient record, and the electronic medical record remains subject to propagation of copied materials that are incorrect—indeed, it may be easier to copy incorrect data in an electronic medical record because of the ease of copy and paste.

Certainly, the electronic medical record can be a useful tool in ensuring that evidence-based medical practice is followed. Indeed, in the Veterans Administration system, where electronic medical records were developed, use of prompts and reminders resulted in higher performance levels.

But perhaps the biggest flaw in electronic medical records is the general inability of the systems to which they belong to communicate with one another. If a patient has an electronic medical record in one office where he or she obtains care, the system of which this medical record is a part may not communicate with a system containing a similar record in another medical practice. This duplication of efforts adds cost to the health care system and increases the potential for errors; there is no opportunity to reconcile information available in the two records. Further, inclusion of paper records into an electronic medical record generally occurs by saving an electronic copy of the paper record in the patient's chart. Such a record might include valuable information, but practically speaking, it is unusable.

Additionally, the electronic record has made it hard to speak with a patient without looking at the computer screen. This is not good for the doctor/patient relationship, yet a greater dependence on the electronic medical record is taking more and more time from the provider-patient encounter and robbing providers of the time necessary to do what they do best: talk with and examine their patients.

While some of these problems were fostered by concurrent, simultaneous development of different systems of electronic medical records that did not have a common source code, they have been aggravated by issues around compliance and patient privacy that are intended to protect patient privacy, but sometimes can confound and complicate treatment. And as "meaningful use" of electronic health care records was introduced as part of the ACA, unfortunately, neither a requirement for different types of electronic medical records to work together nor required use of unique identifiers for patients were included. These changes would have accelerated data acquisition, and data querying abilities exponentially. It is not too late to mandate such policies.

Data acquisition methods for collecting and distilling mean-ingful phenotypic patient information that could be joined with biometric and genomic information are being developed. In the near future, creation and acquisition of large cross-cultural demographic and genomic information will have a major impact on prevention and the use of much more targeted—and less risky—treatments. These innovations should stimulate the econ-omy, improve patient care and outcomes, and overall, drive down health care costs.

What To Do

Several relatively simple steps can be taken to help achieve the promise of electronic medical records. Perhaps the first step is to simply acknowledge that medicine is in a period of such complexity that, without machine learning and cloud-based solutions, no one provider can possibly know all the information necessary to effectively manage all aspects of a disease. Second would be to acknowledge the overall goal of technology: to harness it so that it enhances patients' experiences with health care systems and improves the value of care they receive. Achieving these goals requires several steps.

First, common standards that allow for interactivity of patient records that are derived from different electronic medical record systems should be developed and required to be installed by the medical record system manufacturers. This would dramatically improve interoperability of these records and allow for synchronization of information across medical records as it becomes available. Not only would this improve providers' ability to rely on the data in these records, but it would prevent errors and reduce redundant use of tests. Recent medication changes would be recorded and distributed, as would lab results, so that providers need not reorder a test that had recently been completed.

Second, the medical record should follow the patient and not be restricted to a health care system or office. Cloud-based computing, already available today, that is secure and compliant with the Health Insurance Portability and Accountability Act (HIPAA) and the Federal Information Security and Management Act (FISMA), could allow this to happen. Then, in addition to information from other direct health care providers, information from ancillary providers such as pharmacists could be included. The tremendous thing about the advent of computer order entry by physicians was that it prevented medication interactions; the problem with it is that it is currently limited to care provided within a single system. Cloud-based computing could make this data—as well as data obtained from individual monitoring devices and other inputs that patients might want to include (such as information on dietary habits, exercise, blood glucose levels)—available to all of a patient's health care providers. The obstacle to immediate implementation is not the technology itself, but the need to comply with regulations and to develop partnerships with organizations that have the technological capacity and the desire to use that capacity to benefit patients.

Third, while the above changes would make electronic health care records accessible and data-rich, they would still be information-poor. To address this problem, common templates and data fields should be used, and algorithms applied to determine patient disease trajectories. Indeed, one could imagine a "smart" system—perhaps not unlike one that Amazon might use to anticipate another book you might like after you ordered a first one—that might use the previously mentioned sensors to monitor patients' health status (for instance, determining whether their glucose is getting out of control or there is evidence of an impending asthma attack) and send them instructions when they are believed to be vulnerable. Similarly, such records could anticipate when a patient is running out of a medication and could both confirm that the patient wants to continue receiving the medication and could facilitate the ordering (and perhaps delivery) of the refill.

Fourth, patient-reported outcomes should be incorporated into the medical record—they should be collected electronically on a regular basis to track disease progression and reported with the simplicity found in reporting the contents of a cereal box. For instance, in the case of knee replacement, systems can be developed to identify the level of pain and disability that knee pain is causing, identify the impact of several different types of interventions on that pain and disability, and track those changes over time. This information would help a patient like John identify when the best time might be to have knee replacement surgery—it could answer, for a patient with his sociodemographic characteristics—what kind of outcomes might be anticipated for different interventions, and whether he might be best served by acting quickly or waiting to pursue knee replacement surgery.

Finally, medical records should be able to provide a consolidated, simple, and relevant summary of a patient's recent history, recent changes, current medications, and reasons for the visit. They should also include information on the patient's personal life: whether the patient has experienced a recent stressor, whether the patient has recently moved, and even whether the patient is a physician. The technology to do this already exists. For instance, retail service companies such as credit card providers contact a customer, name him or her correctly, use the proper salutation, and can know what recent transactions were (and even whether they were "out of character," making the company intervene to ensure the transactions were intended). In health care, we need to apply such existing technologies to better engage with our patients.

Characteristics of current and future methods for data collection and use are shown in **Figure 2** on the next page.

As is often the case, the challenge in realizing the promise of medical records is in the coordination of efforts. Much as the doctor, nurse, and support staff in a hospital need to work together to help a particular patient, information technology must be coordinated and integrated into the work flow to help achieve that same goal.

Medicine can and must learn from other service industries, the minimum of which is to treat a patient with courtesy and respect. Well-designed electronic medical records must become a facilitator of these efforts, a partner in the care of our patients and their families. Already, several other industries have started to enter the new economy of health and health care by collecting patient data, monitoring patient outcomes, and analyzing them for the purposes of managing the overall population.

Figure 2. Characteristics of current and future methods for data collection and use.

	Current	**Future**
Data collection	• Paper • Repeat entry of same data • Provided by patient • Stagnant and cross-sectional • Stored in files	• Electronic with personal sensors • Eliminates redundancy • Augmented by electronics • Fluid and longitudinal • Cloud-based, secure, and accessible
Data uses	• Billing • Focused on what happened • Retrospective and reactive • Stand-alone systems • Separated from other data • Informed by provider review of available data	• Health management with data analytics • Focused on results with transparent reporting • Anticipatory and proactive • Encompassing all health-care encounters • Integrated with other data • Informed by data on all health encounters, other data, data analytics, and clinical support

Chapter 3

The Visit—Patient Perspective

John Alvarez is a 52-year-old Hispanic male who owns a small chain of convenience stores in southern Vermont. John is active, happy, and has been married for 32 years. He has four children, all of whom are now out of the house. He prides himself on the professionalism and customer-friendly attitude of his convenience store employees. While by virtue of the job, many of his employees are in their late teens or early twenties, he has created a customer service "onboarding" program for new hires. The training—which only takes about 30 minutes—trains the clerks to be respectful and patient, to always ask if the customer needs anything else, to say "thank you for coming in" when the customer leaves, and to look each customer in the eye.

John is due for a routine physical exam. He hasn't had one in a few years—mostly because things were getting kind of busy at work. But at his wife's insistence, John makes an appointment. They have good health insurance through the company (and John is proud to offer health insurance to all his employees, regardless of whether they work full time or part time), and John knew he was probably due for a "50-year checkup."

Before going to the appointment, John and his wife, Anita, discuss his health. Anita is concerned that John has put on about 20 pounds in the last few years—he has an old football injury that was keeping him from exercising. She is also scared: a friend of theirs who had not gotten a screening colonoscopy at age 50 had been diagnosed with colon cancer when he turned 54. And while his case was straightforward, he relayed several times how his oncologist had told him that, had he had the screening colonoscopy, he could have avoided several hospital stays, a surgery, a temporary colostomy, and three rounds of chemotherapy. Finally, Anita is worried about John's capacity for intimacy; over the past few years, their sex life has dwindled — just when the kids had moved out of the house, it seemed. She knows there are medications that can help, and she also knows that sometimes sexual dysfunction is a symptom of other health-related issues. So Anita helps John prepare for the visit: she writes down important questions for the doctor, and she helps him with the health history forms that were sent to him for completion prior to the visit.

John arrives at the appointment with his papers in hand. He is told that the doctor is running late, so he waits for about 30 minutes. A woman who does not introduce herself calls his name and asks him to follow her. She instructs him to take off his shoes, and weighs him and records his height. She then tells him to sit down and open his mouth. As he does, she concurrently sticks a thermometer in his mouth and places a blood pressure cuff on his arm. "Uncross your legs," she says, pointing to a poster on the wall that explains that having crossed legs during a blood pressure reading could distort the accuracy of the measurement. They wait a minute in silence while she fills out some paperwork. "OK," she says, handing him a backless gown, "take your clothes off, put this on, and sit on the table."

Fifteen minutes later a white-coated man comes into the room, holding a computer. He looks at John, and says, "Hi, I'm Dr. Glickly. You must be Mr." — he looks down at the computer screen — "Alvarez. Good to meet you. What can I do for you today?"

John tells him he is there for a checkup. The doctor asks if he had any specific concerns, and John says, "Yes, a few — I raised them on the forms you sent."

"We never get time to look those over," Dr. Glickly says. "Just tell me what they are."

John tells him about the weight gain and that he thought he was due for a colonoscopy, but he doesn't feel comfortable talking about the intimacy issue. Dr. Glickly takes notes and stares at the computer screen.

"OK," he says. "Lie back—I'm going to feel your belly."

Dr. Glickly palpates John's stomach, listens to John's heart and lungs, and taps on his knees and the inside of his elbows.

"OK," Dr. Glickly says, turning his back to John and typing on the computer. "We'll get you scheduled for a colonoscopy. And I'm going to give you an ACE inhibitor—your blood pressure is a little high. Also, we need to do some blood tests—the front desk will schedule those for you." He gets up from his chair, holding the computer, and looks over the raised screen. "Anything else I can do for you?"

"No, thanks. I'm good," John says.

"OK, then. See you later." And Dr. Glickly walks out of the room, looking down at the computer screen.

How We Got Here

Health care delivery is a complex combination of science and art, in many cases heavily emphasizing the art. The process entails collecting and integrating subjective information (what the patient thinks is going on), objective information (including patient vital signs and findings from the physical exam), and research (which guides physicians on what tests to perform when and which interventions to make to decrease the spread of disease). Part of the art of medicine is the assimilation of these different streams of information in a way that helps patients maintain their health.

But over the past half century, health care delivery has ceded some of its art form to technology. Technological advances have contributed to the effectiveness of health care delivery in some areas while offering the potential to overdiagnose in others.

The abilities to locate possible disease states through diagnostic imaging and tests and to intervene with "minimally invasive" procedures to address those supposed diseases can disrupt efforts to just provide good, responsive care.

As discussed in the last chapter, adoption of the evolving electronic medical record has been a double-edged sword for health care providers. Electronic medical records are certainly easier for others to read, they can make records easier to find, and they can, in some instances, provide real-time reminders so that health care providers can adhere to evidence-based medical practices and avoid potential dangers (such as drug interactions). But sometimes they can interfere with the doctor-patient relationship and cause more problems than they solve.

One of the key problems with trying to integrate technology into the health care delivery setting is using it appropriately. Too often, electronic medical records are simply used to ensure better billing practices and document aspects of the encounter that might not be related to health or health care. The records can encourage providers to do a more thorough "review of systems" or to palpate another body system, in part to improve the thoroughness of care provided to patients, but also in part to generate higher billing levels. Generally, reimbursement is contingent on a particular number of systems being examined and the subjective complexity of the problem being treated. So, in an effort to maximize revenues, many health care systems will emphasize doing more services and collecting more data, often more than they emphasize collecting the right data. And Mr. Alvarez's case shows us that.

In the example, Mr. Alvarez's body was properly monitored and examined. He obtained treatment for a new finding—hypertension. His vital signs were collected, entered into the electronic medical record, and could undoubtedly be later reviewed in graphic form to, for instance, monitor the responsiveness of his hypertension to the new medication.

But in the encounter, Mr. Alvarez was lost. The time he spent preparing for the appointment was wasted—the paper forms were not read or integrated into the medical record or interview. The limited time he had with the doctor was seemingly wasted on data collection that was largely irrelevant to Mr. Alvarez's primary concerns. And while he will get additional testing—including the colonoscopy—what he is to do with the information gleaned from that testing is not clear.

Most importantly, Mr. Alvarez was not able to get one of his primary concerns addressed or even discussed; it simply was not made relevant to the interview or exam. And while patients have difficulties discussing problems of intimacy with physicians—particularly new ones with whom they have not developed a relationship—physicians have their own challenges discussing certain topics, including important ones like intimacy, stress and depression, and end-of-life planning. Too, although many providers may regret the intrusion of the electronic medical record, they are reassured that the data collected through its use will eventually be helpful in achieving the "meaningful use" criteria outlined in the Affordable Care Act.

So health care delivery has evolved into a chaotic and bureaucratic business with systems prioritized above patients. Currently, health care delivery is neither patient nor physician centered. Physicians are expensive assets—their time is valuable and should be used as efficiently as possible. Their value is really only derived from the benefits they convey, including the knowledge and skills acquired through a minimum of a decade of training and demonstrated through board certification and maintenance processes that exceed requirements of any other profession. Though airline pilots continuously train to make air travel safe, they fly in planes with standard features and autopilot capabilities; the planes can fly themselves. While some aspects of what providers do can be replaced with technology, human courtesy, compassion, and customer service are irreplaceable characteristics that providers must retain and demonstrate as necessary and critical components of comprehensive care provided to patients and their families. And although the patient-centered care movement is taking hold, it is young. A friend of ours with cancer who recently encountered challenges within the health care system told us that he knew what patient-centered care really means: it means that the patient better be in the center of and in charge of his care, because no one else is.

What To Do

Unfortunately, encounters with the health care system like the one Mr. Alvarez had are not uncommon. Inappropriate use of technology, excessive focus on pathology, inadequate time with the provider, and lack of focus on understanding and meeting patients' needs are reparable. We just need to set up the system to get the incentives right in order to promote their being done correctly.

First, the provision of care should be designed around the patient: patient needs, concerns, and convenience should drive all aspects of care delivery. Health care delivery systems should value the patient's time — the time spent in preparation for, at, and after the appointment. Here, integration of technology should focus on the patient's convenience. Might Mr. Alvarez have completed the forms online, through a web portal that downloaded his information into the medical record, identified his concerns for the doctor to immediately address, and tracked such information over time to determine whether Mr. Alvarez's problems were being resolved? Further, validated instruments that screen for common health problems, such as depression or intimacy issues, could be used to highlight areas for the physician to review. The use of technology in this way would have aligned Dr. Glickly's and Mr. Alvarez's interests. Instead of looking over a computer screen to make inquiries of Mr. Alvarez, Dr. Glickly could have been looking at the computer screen with Mr. Alvarez to discuss the reasons Mr. Alvarez was seeking consultation.

Clearly, alignment of incentives to maximize the value that a patient obtains from care is critical to improving the effectiveness and efficiency of health care delivery. Imagine for a moment that the goal of health care delivery was to promote health and to work with patients to maximize the joy they derive from life by helping keep them healthy and happy. The focus of activities around this goal would be to work with the patient to identify and try to meet health goals. The relationship would be more of a coaching relationship that incorporates the subjective (what the patient wants and says he needs), the objective (what the lab results and the scales tell the doctor and patient), and research (information on what works and what the side effects of interventions are). Interventions should be predicated on what the patient values (whether any side effects are worth the intervention) and informed by data on outcomes that allow patients to make informed decisions about their health.

This kind of work would be collective and shared between the patient and the health care team. It would be focused on what the patient wants. It would be technologically savvy, capturing elements that enhance the patient's ability to meet his or her goals. It would be shared across a treatment team, with members who might have different expertise that would be tapped, when required, to help the patient live a healthy life. Reimbursement would not revolve around documenting whether a part of the body was palpated, but on whether the patient was achieving his or her health goals; it would not be based on the illness burden that patients carried, but on their ability to successfully reduce those burdens, over time.

Most importantly, the patient would be central to care. Patients could reach members of the health care team through a variety of means and not always in person. Testing could be done at the patient's convenience and integrated into the medical record for collaborative, review and monitoring. Health care choices — such as whether to diet or exercise or begin taking a new medication — would be informed and in most cases, would not require an immediate decision, but one that could be mulled over, so the patient could benefit from the input of other people the decision might impact. A comparison of provider-centered and patient-centered care is provided in **Figure 3**.

Figure 3. A comparison of provider-centered and patient-centered care.

	Provider-centered	Patient-centered
Access	In person at the provider's office	Through whatever mechanism is most convenient for the patient, including home-based electronic visits
Care provision	Focused on what the provider can do	Focused on meeting the health-care needs of the patient and using technology to anticipate those needs
Decision model	Provider knows best	Informed choice to match decisions to patient's goals and values
Belief system	More is better	Avoid overuse, misuse, and underuse
Goal	Address illness	Monitor and improve health in an ongoing fashion
Payment	Fee-for-service	Capitated

Finally, technology could determine the value of the care provided and the value created by anticipated interventions. By analyzing and displaying data collected from other patients who have faced similar decisions, patients might be able to determine probable outcomes for patients like themselves — for instance, patients of the same gender with a similar age, level of disability, and list of treatment priorities. This kind of analysis and transparency regarding the outcomes of prior patients treated at the institution where the patient is seeking care could help patients determine whether to have an intervention and — by comparing results from several health care providers — where to have the intervention done. Eventually, health care organizations might use this information to both advertise what they do well and inexpensively, and to consider which health care options to offer patients. For instance, if an organization cannot clearly demonstrate a similarly high value in treatment of diabetics, the organization might consider letting other health care systems provide such care and focus on the care they can most effectively and efficiently provide.

Technology holds tremendous promise for health care. But it needs to be directed so that patients are the greatest beneficiaries of its use and so that, like any health care intervention, it can be used in the most efficient and effective manner for promoting health..

Chapter 4

The Visit—Provider Perspective

Frederick Landesman is a 52-year-old family practice physician who has been in the same small group practice with four other physicians, three nurse practitioners, two medical assistants, an office manager, and a secretary ever since he completed his residency 22 years ago. He joined the practice as a junior associate, and he worked hard to pay off more than $100,000 of accumulated college and medical school debt. Even though that was a lot of money, he felt lucky; he had been able to attend state schools, whereas some physicians he knew had attended private colleges and medical schools and had racked up triple his debt. During his three-year residency, he had moonlighted in a local emergency room to be able to afford to pay off his student loans without it growing somewhat exponentially (which is what happens when the interest expenses are "capitalized"). His residency was an exhausting three years—capping an 11-year path to becoming a board-certified family practice physician, a career he had dreamed of since he was 12. And while he recalled those wearying years with fondness—they included his marriage, the births of his two sons, and tremendously stimulating learning experiences that he loved and at which he excelled, having graduated in the top 5 percent of his medical school class—on reflection, he's not sure he would do it again.

Fred pursued a medical career for two reasons. First, like many he encountered in medical school, he had a close family member who was chronically ill. His grandmother, who watched him after school while he was in elementary school, had diabetes, atherosclerotic vascular disease, and congestive heart failure. He saw quite intimately how fragile and dependent she was on a carefully monitored medical regimen even when she was only about 50. He also saw how random changes in her routine — whether due to her doctor relocating, her being hospitalized to get a knee replacement, or her forgetting to get a prescription refilled — dramatically and adversely impacted her life and resulted in emergency room visits, hospitalizations, or her just feeling lousy. Her somewhat premature death was precipitated by an adverse drug reaction that landed her in the hospital and from which she never really recovered. He vowed to become a doctor so he could take better care of people like his grandmother. Second, he liked helping people, a feeling that grew during his residency years. Although the residency was long and difficult, he still felt incredible compassion for his patients and enjoyed getting to know them.

Fred went into family practice because he knew that there was a great need for primary care physicians and that the research showed that greater availability of primary care physicians was associated with better patient satisfaction, better outcomes, and lower health care costs. He had imagined having a personal and relaxed practice, where the door was always open, where he had time to attend to his patients' needs, and where he could actively participate in helping his patients' families grow older.

His practice started out that way; he enjoyed his colleagues, and they shared the same philosophy and goals. But over the last 15 years, it seemed like the practice had gotten more and more complex — he and his partners would jokingly refer to the third person in the room with them and their patient: the insurer. Over the years, it seemed to Fred that insurers and regulators occupied more and more space in the exam room, and it took more and more time to address insurers' needs — time and space that were extracted from that previously shared with patients. First, there were quality controls designed to reduce hospital admissions, then controls on the medications he prescribed, and then suggestions on the tests that needed to be done. Finally, the medical record, which did not seem to help with care so much as it took up even more space in the patient encounter, seemingly robbed Fred of his most valuable diagnostic instruments: his ears, eyes, and touch — his ability to listen, see, and examine.

Fred was a pretty conservative family practice physician who tried to take the time to inform patients about their treatment options. He mostly recommended watchful waiting, waiting a bit before getting a test or a procedure done, knowing that the good old tincture of time, combined with rest, is a pretty effective healer. But the combination of erroneous Internet information and advertising by special interest groups made his conservatism harder and harder to maintain. His patients were reading one-sided information about the latest test or intervention and would then want to get it. He was appalled at the mobile full-body CT scanning companies that would scan his (insured) patients and give them a report that found all sorts of irregularities, often normal variants, which they would then bring to him in a terrified state. He spent hours reviewing those reports, ones that often noted "the possibility" or "the potential for development" for one abnormality or another. And while he counseled his patients about the general ineffectiveness of screening for diseases in populations that were at low risk for those diseases, they were still worried.

Having just returned a call to a patient to check on the effectiveness of a medication change, he sat at his desk and wondered how it might be different. It was six thirty in the evening, he had been at the office since seven that morning, and he had seen 30 patients — 15 in the morning session and 15 in the afternoon — being able to spend approximately 12 minutes with each one. He tried to keep up with recording his notes during the encounter, but the typing and focus on the computer kept him from connecting with his patients. He had another hour of work at least and was going to miss dinner with his family again. He figured that half—maybe three-quarters—of the patients he had seen today did not need to be seen in person, but, as his office manager chided him every time he returned a phone call, "insurance doesn't pay for phone calls, and phone calls don't pay bills."

"Surely there must be a better way," he thought.

How We Got Here

Primary care has long been the backbone of health care across the world. Primary care providers serve critical roles in health care delivery: they monitor the health of the patients they serve, they are frequently the first contact that patients have when they become ill, they manage patients' care, they help patients understand treatment options, and they help them arrive at the best path forward—whether that decision is around getting a test, pursuing an intervention, or considering end-of-life care. Primary care providers have long acted as trusted navigators to make the health care system work for patients and their families.

Such navigation helps patients obtain high-quality, low-cost care. Where there are more primary care providers, patients have greater satisfaction with their care, they sense that care is more readily available to them (even when there are fewer physicians per capita in the marketplace), they use care more efficiently (fewer tests and interventions), they experience lower health care costs, and they often have better health outcomes.

In the United States, it is widely acknowledged that there is a relative paucity of primary care providers. Indeed, frequently, residency positions in primary care fields (such as family practice, pediatrics, and general internal medicine) go unfilled; a relatively large proportion of those positions are filled by foreign medical school graduates because U.S. medical school graduates do not want to practice primary care medicine. In contrast, residencies in some specialties (such as orthopedic surgery, ophthalmology, dermatology, and radiology) are highly sought after, and there are often multiple applicants for a single position.

Studies have identified several reasons why primary care fields are less attractive than specialty care fields. First, primary care specialists seem to have considerably less control over their lives than do physicians in specialty practices, where procedures are often scheduled weeks in advance and providers often act as consultants to pieces of overall care management and are not as engaged in the day-to-day, overall health care needs of their patients. Certainly, both specialists and primary care providers have emergencies, but primary care providers seem to experience more less-urgent ones and they are expected to be available to their own patients. Because younger medical school graduates appear to want to enter fields that have better lifestyles that include predictable hours and more time off, fewer of them are attracted to primary care medicine.

Second, primary care providers seem to have less support than do their specialist counterparts; they tend to have fewer support staff and team members and to act more independently. In part, this is a function of the lack of technology in most primary care practices — when there is no procedure room, operating room, or common need for complex radiographic tests, care can be provided relatively simply, with fewer people. And this support is increasingly important as regulation and oversight of health care processes become progressively more intrusive. Particularly in smaller group practice settings — and over 75 percent of primary care practices are groups of fewer than five physicians — addressing that regulation and oversight can be overwhelming.

Additionally, primary care providers seem to be somewhat less respected than are their specialist colleagues. This is likely because of the slow, accumulating incremental value that primary care providers supply to their patients over time as opposed to the more dramatic and immediate value that specialists provide. Patients are more likely to attribute their pain relief and newfound mobility to the orthopedic surgeon who replaced their knees than they are to attribute their general health and sense of well-being to their primary care physician. And even when a primary care physician does his job exceptionally well — diagnosing a rare disorder or an early cancer, expeditiously arranging for treatment, and extending life — subsequent care is quickly removed from the primary care doctor.

Finally, primary care physicians get paid a lot less than do the highly sought after specialists. While it is true that those specialties have longer residency periods — a typical primary care residency is three years and that for a specialty is four to six years — the financial returns that specialists obtain rapidly warrant the extra couple of years in residency. And given the tremendous amounts of debt that providers incur on their way to board certification (including the high cost of medical education, compounded by the rising cost of undergraduate education), the much higher returns on educational investment make specialty practice that much more attractive.

Efforts to expand the primary care physician workforce have largely been unsuccessful. However, the Affordable Care Act includes several provisions designed to enlarge that workforce, including an increase in reimbursement rates, student loan support, improved insurance for patients, and payments designed to foster the establishment of medical homes that rely more on primary care providers. But such incentives might take decades to become effective, as students now entering medical school will not be available to practice primary care medicine for seven years or so.

What To Do

Several more immediate remedies could work in concert with the provisions of the Affordable Care Act to improve the attractiveness of primary care medicine, enhance patient access to primary care physicians, and improve both the patient and provider experience of primary care encounters.

First, new models of care that distribute more funding to support better primary care encounters are needed. While the Affordable Care Act improves the per-visit reimbursement rate for primary care physicians, that incentive is misguided in two ways. First, while reimbursements per visit are scheduled to improve, the focus on visit-based reimbursements incentivizes more face-to-face care, when substitution of other forms of care provision might be more effective. Indeed, it may be much more convenient and efficient for both the provider and the patient to manage some care interventions by phone, e-mail, home visits, or telemedicine, and each of these methods could be further enhanced by the use of remote sensing. But because reimbursement remains contingent on face-to-face health care interactions, paradoxically, access to care is reduced. When a doctor's schedule is booked with visits, some of which could be managed more effectively in these other ways, it becomes more difficult for patients who need a doctor visit to get that care.

Second, the ACA provides only the most modest increase in payments, one that is not likely to have a great effect on the construct of the physician workforce. While primary care reimbursement might improve more in the future, the financial returns to specialty care practice will still dwarf those accruing to medical students who pursue primary care.

A better model would place the primary care physician at the center of patient care provision and fairly pay the provider on the basis of keeping a cohort of patients well and out of the health care system. Such a model would encourage primary care providers to use alternative forms of communication (other than face-to-face) with their patients and allow primary care providers to perform office procedures that are within the realm of their competencies, instead of always referring patients to expensive specialists. For procedures that primary care physicians could not safely perform, a shared decision-making process that ensures choices are consistent with patients' values, and that patients really want and need a particular diagnostic or procedural intervention, could be conducted in the primary care provider's office. For specialty care, the primary care provider could use a narrow network of providers who are able to transparently demonstrate that the care they provide is appropriate, high-value care.

For elective health care procedures, "high-value care" can be defined as a high ratio of patient outcomes and satisfaction divided by total costs of care over time (for instance, including all care provided in the 60 days after a procedure). While the costs of care during an inpatient admission do not show much variation within a diagnosis-related-group (DRG), research has found substantial variation in the costs of care that follow discharge. This variation appears to reflect practice habits and does not appear to be related to health care outcomes. Too often, these practice patterns are driven by the infrastructure put into place to sustain the system financially. We have a health care delivery system that was built on an outmoded approach to health and health care, one that has not adapted to advances in anesthesia operative techniques and new technologies. But we sustain this infrastructure because of the financial obligations that were taken on as it was built.

Indeed, substitution of lower-cost care — such as home health care that is supported by using wearable sensors, distance-technology, and computer-based algorithms — for additional time in the hospital can save substantial money for the patient and the health care system without adversely impacting health outcomes. Frequently, such substitution also provides more convenient and better care for patients and their families.

Some of the cost savings that accrue to insurers from primary care physicians' referral to high-value care providers should go back to the primary care practices and the communities they serve. One could imagine block grants for communities that keep themselves well. They could use those for immunization programs, drug benefits, or wellness in the form of a public pool that would benefit the whole community. Indeed, by using evidence-based referral practices and block grants from saved medical resources to direct their patients to the highest value care and to enhance the health of the communities in which they practice, primary care providers would be providing a service to their patients and to society in general.

Clearly, some patients might want to obtain care outside of the evidence-based, narrow, high-value care network, and they should be able to. Here, too, primary care providers should provide — and be reimbursed for — shared decision-making processes. But insurers should partner with primary care physicians to steer patients to only high-value care proceduralists through benefits design. Should patients elect to obtain care outside of the evidence-based high-value network, their out-of-pocket costs should be higher to cover the difference, so as to help defray costs that are objectively anticipated to cost more, but are not associated with better outcomes.

As shown in **Figure 4** on the next page, primary care provider offices should serve as the community control centers that allow multiple forms of care access, help maintain the health of their patient populations, help patients make informed decisions, help guide patients to the demonstrably highest value care possible, and coordinate patient care. Funds unleashed through cost savings generated by primary care physicians' augmented roles could give primary care providers the support — in the form of traditional medical assistants and even scribes — needed to provide personal, attentive service that is not impeded, but rather enhanced by new technology partners. Electronic medical records should include modules that can be used to identify

Figure 4. A comparison of current and future primary and specialty physician roles.

	Current role and function	Future role and function
Primary care provider	• Works to address illness • Manages across wide spectrum of complexity • Relatively underpaid, based on fee-for-service • Accessed for primary care, makes referrals • Uses patient demand to manage care • Effectiveness measured on quality of care given to particular patients • Inadequate numbers	• Works to maintain health • Manages a narrower spectrum of complexity by using midlevel providers and technology • Higher paid, based on population health management • Source for shared decision-making processes, including best-value care • Uses technology to anticipate care needs • Effectiveness measured on health of the community served • Adequate numbers
Specialty care provider	• Redundant evaluation • Fee-for-service reimbursement • Supplier-induced demand generates services • Too many, making too much money	• More efficient use with less reevaluation • Reimbursed as a carve-out • Shared decision-making by primary care limits supplier-induced demand • Fewer, making more reasonable salaries

patient preferences regarding care options. These would integrate proceduralist-specific outcomes with detailed information on health care trajectories that could be used to identify outcomes for patients with particular demographic characteristics, thereby answering the question, "How would this procedure impact a patient like me?"

Over time, practice as a primary care physician would become more supported, respected, and financially successful. With increased competition for fewer procedures, one might anticipate that rapid increases in the reimbursement for specialists might lessen and become based on outcomes and not on lobbying power. Then more medical students might pursue primary care practices. In all, this redistribution of responsibilities should curtail growth of health care costs, improve the health of the population, and improve the newly supported supply of primary care providers.

Chapter 5

The Tests

Marie is a 49-year-old homemaker and the mother of four children, only one of whom, a junior in high school, is still living at home. Marie's husband, Jim, is a successful businessman. They are supportive of their community — Jim serves as Chair of the school board, Marie is the primary community liaison of the women's fellowship at the Congregational Church.

Marie and Jim have excellent insurance, and being health conscious, Marie makes sure everyone in the family has an annual physical exam. Prior to last year, Marie worked out about five times a week, but this year, with the twins going off to separate colleges, her work at the women's fellowship, and her time volunteering at the food shelf, she did not seem to have time to exercise more than once or twice a week. She'd put on about 10 pounds, and she was worried that her new primary care physician would be concerned about her health. The primary care physician whom she had seen for 25 years had just retired, and her physical exam was scheduled with a new family practice physician who had recently completed residency.

In the doctor's office, Marie completed a number of forms, and many questions seemed to be similar to the screening forms she'd completed and sent in two weeks before. Aside from the weight gain, Marie felt healthy, except for a kind of dull pain just to the left of her lower back that she'd had since she had slipped on the ice about two months ago. She was a little anxious about meeting the new physician, but she recognized the nurse who'd taken her vital signs before the appointment as the same person who had been taking them for years.

After the initial information intake, Marie sat in the exam room in a gown. Dr. Jefferson came in, introduced himself, and reviewed her past medical history with her (which was pretty sparse, except for the pregnancies, when she'd had gestational diabetes and a cesarean section with the twins). As Marie was nearing 50, Dr. Jefferson told her that she should get several tests, including a screening colonoscopy, a mammogram, and screening for hypercholesterolemia and diabetes. Also, Dr. Jefferson recommended an MRI of her back, given the pain, and a sleep study, as she'd indicated on the screening forms that she'd been snoring more lately.

A month later Marie returned to see Dr. Jefferson, after having completed the recommended tests. Dr. Jefferson seemed a bit rushed, but he noted that she had slightly high LDL cholesterol levels ("the bad kind of cholesterol," he'd said). Further, her nonfasting blood glucose level was 105, slightly above normal. In addition, the sleep study had indicated "micro apneic spells," which Dr. Jefferson told her were consistent with sleep apnea. The MRI had shown "T2 weighted evidence of swelling that was indicative of modest herniation with mild nerve compression at the L5–S1 level." The colonoscopy was normal, but the mammogram showed "microcalcifications that should be followed over time." Finally, Dr. Jefferson told her that with a blood pressure of 126/84, she was considered "prehypertensive," and he recommended starting an antihypertension drug.

Marie was a bit overwhelmed, but Dr. Jefferson had seemingly already set out a course of action. He'd ordered a lipid-lowering medication, scheduled her for a fasting glucose study, had a continuous positive airway pressure machine on hand for her to take home, and had scheduled a repeat mammography in two months. He asked her if she'd like him to refer her to a spine surgeon to address the possible disc herniation.

That night at home, Marie discussed the encounter with her *husband. She was surprised that, with all the testing, she only had to pay a total of $60 in copayments, although the bills totaled about $6,000.*

"Maybe you should get a second opinion," Jim said.

Two weeks later Marie did just that. Another primary care physician, Dr. Gilbert, suggested that she restart exercising and watch her diet. She did, and within about two months she found that she slept better without snoring, her back did not hurt, and her glucose, lipid levels, and blood pressure had all returned to normal, without medications.

Marie obtained a follow-up mammography six months later, and as the microcalcifications had not changed, she obtained a breast biopsy that was negative for breast cancer.

How We Got Here

As we have indicated before, providers in the health care system are paid on a fee-for-service basis. In non-health care industries, this type of reimbursement model is called "piecework." Workers are paid according to the number of items they produce—the more they produce, the more money they make. The challenge with this type of reimbursement is that the quality of the product might suffer as workers strive to produce more of them, unless there are objective measures of quality.

In health care, providers generally are not responsible for the additional health care resources that their actions consume. There is an old adage that physicians consume 20 percent of the health care dollar, but direct how the other 80 percent is spent. And multiple studies have demonstrated that providers generally have no idea how much the additional services they order cost. There are huge opportunities to curtail health care spending with regard to diagnostic testing and ample evidence that excessive testing not only does not help patients, but can actually hurt them.

Perhaps not widely understood is that all health care tests have a "false-positive" rate; this occurs when an initial test result is abnormal, but on repeat testing comes back normal. For any of a variety of reasons, the first test's results generated an abnormal reading. Tests are designed to minimize this possibility—this is part of the reason normal test ranges are relatively wide—but false positives can occur about 5 percent of the time. And false positives are more common when the test is performed on a low-risk population. Indeed, when HIV testing was recommended as a requirement for obtaining a marriage license in the 1990s, an analysis revealed that many more positive tests would be false positives than true positives because the population being considered for widespread testing—young, heterosexual people who were intending to get married—was at a very low risk of having HIV.

A similar problem occurs with most other testing. Radiographic tests (x-rays, CAT scans, MRI scans, and ultrasounds) have become so sophisticated that they can identify very small "abnormalities"—abnormalities that many providers believe might either go away without intervention or just might be a variant of "normal." The challenge to providers is to use this extremely accurate and yet expensive technology wisely and sparingly. As can be seen from Marie's case, overuse of such technology not only costs money, but also may create unnecessary worry—or real harm—and lead to too much unnecessary attention being given to normal variants. In particular, radiographic precision has exceeded medicine's understanding of the natural trajectory of illness.

In part because of medicolegal issues, interpretation of much testing is intentionally vague; readers of radiological test or sleep apnea tests may "overcall" disease states, creating pseudodisease states, because of a fear of later lawsuits if they "underread" the test. But this tendency to have low thresholds for abnormal readings places an obligation on the provider who ordered the test to act. This means that, in response to overdiagnosis, providers will often order additional tests, schedule interventions, and possibly even recommend biopsies, as in this case, which further causes fear, anxiety, and harm potential. Prescription medications themselves are not without risk; as is shown in Marie's case, behavioral changes sometimes can effectively improve symptoms while avoiding untoward medication side effects or unanticipated interactions with other ongoing treatments. Unfortunately, when a potpourri of providers is involved in a particular case, there is more opportunity for unnecessary testing, more diagnoses, and greater use of medications. Too often, this lack of care coordination makes a patient's life more and more complicated, and more and more dominated by medical concerns. Further, the more complex the treatment protocol, the more opportunities there are for treatment errors or harms, including treatment mistakes, drug interactions, and miscommunication between providers.

Additionally, as shown in this case, harried providers often have a propensity to use medical interventions as opposed to conservative interventions to address problems. Sometimes more conservative interventions that involve "watchful waiting" can be more effective; however, more conservative interventions also can require more provider engagement and time, in part because patients have come to expect some kind of intervention to "fix" whatever finding is revealed by a test. It is often more expeditious to simply write a prescription that might treat the numbers or the symptoms than it is to engage the patient in a discussion about a behavioral-based lifestyle change, which may have a far more lasting impact; and patients sometimes are more satisfied with a pill than with a recommendation for lifestyle change.

One problem with testing is that any identified abnormalities, like the microcalcifications found on Marie's mammogram, require follow-up, sometimes for extensive periods. Another, perhaps more lasting problem, is that "abnormal" test results create labels, which can have lasting—and sometimes negative—impacts on patients, employers, and insurers.

In sum, testing costs a lot of money, both immediately and in the longer term, as costs from repeat testing, pharmaceutical treatments, or additional procedures are used to address abnormal test results. Once again we see several factors aligning to increase the costs—and likely decrease the effectiveness—of health-services delivery. Physicians, who might be concerned about malpractice or simply afraid to miss something, might be predisposed to order more tests and to follow up on them with additional tests and interventions. Patients actually pay little of the testing bill, and they may be reassured by normal test results. In addition, patients may be demanding of action should even mildly "abnormal" or variant results be found. And the financial incentives for doing more testing are clear. While, by law, physicians and group practices are precluded from having investment interests in freestanding testing centers, many physician practices generate substantial additional revenues from doing testing and plain x-rays in their own offices; and hospitals that own physician practices also generate considerable portions of their overall revenues providing radiographic and testing services.

What To Do

Once again, one of the solutions to the potential overuse seen when providers order laboratory or radiographic tests is to align economic incentives. If capitated or global budget mechanisms were in place, so that testing represented a cost center instead of a profit center, overuse of testing would likely decrease. However, underuse of testing can also be problematic; often such tests are indicated and needed. So, how does the system design a method that ensures needed tests are completed, but unneeded ones are not?

As was shown in the RAND health insurance experiment that examined the impact of higher copayments on health care service utilization, leaving choice of services to consumers alone is not necessarily a good idea. When consumers had more incentives to reduce utilization, they were as likely to decrease utilization of high-value services as low-value services. In a similar vein, should providers bear more of the costs of testing — as would be the case in a capitated reimbursement system — they may have similar reactions, foregoing care that patients value because it is expensive.

The best approach is to consider each test independently and to determine ahead of time what actions patients and providers might take if an abnormal test result is found. If they would take no action in response to the test result, the test should not be done, regardless of whether it is indicated. This was illustrated when a large national health system decided to make a big push to complete screening colonoscopies every 10 years on patients who were age 50 or older. Success in achieving this goal would be publicly reported as a performance measure, and as performance measure results were linked to administrator bonuses, there was considerable administrative pressure to complete the colonoscopies.

Two facilities in the system were identified as being poor performers on the colonoscopy measure, and this precipitated a review of the patients who should have gotten colonoscopies based on the indications, but who did not. There were five such patients: two had terminal cancer, two refused to get the test, and one was a frail 95-year-old who, providers felt, was more likely to suffer adverse effects from the colonoscopy and even if a cancer was found, likely would not be able to tolerate the treatment.

So blind adherence to testing protocols, in this case, would have been inappropriate given patients' current medical conditions, would have overridden patient preferences, or would have exposed patients to unnecessary risk.

What was not evaluated in the study was the number of patients who did get the colonoscopy but who, because of their own preferences, illness burden, or age, might have not planned to take action should the colonoscopy have found bowel cancer. Those perhaps, were a far larger number, and their colonoscopies not only cost the health care system considerable resources, but also put those patients at unnecessary risk (colonoscopies have a small but real risk of perforation of the colon, adverse effects from the anesthetic given, and even death). Similar risks are embedded in other screening or diagnostic interventions—including biopsies; therefore, to prevent unnecessary risk exposure, clarity about what would be done, should the diagnostic test reveal the need for further intervention, should be accomplished before the test is completed.

This case and discussion suggest four steps that are necessary to take before a test is completed. First, the person to whom the test is offered should be at some degree of risk of having the illness that the test is designed to identify. If there is no—or very little—risk of the patient having that illness, the likelihood of a false-positive test is greater and the predictive value of the test is poor. Second, the patient should be able to tolerate the test, and the benefits of the test must outweigh the risks. If, because of illness burden or frailty, the test itself poses a significant risk to the patient, the patient should not be subjected to the test. Third, there should be, prior to the procedure, agreement that some specified action would be taken if the test turns out positive. Here too, patient illness burden or frailty might come into play; the patient might be well enough to tolerate the test, but not well enough to tolerate definitive treatment should the test indicate an abnormality. In that case, completing the test is futile and a waste of scarce resources. Finally, the patient should, after being informed of the risks, benefits, and anticipated responses to a positive test result, want to have the test completed. If the patient does not want the test completed, the patient should not be subjected to pressures to have the test. These steps are shown in **Figure 5**.

Figure 5. Process for deciding whether or not to get a medical test.

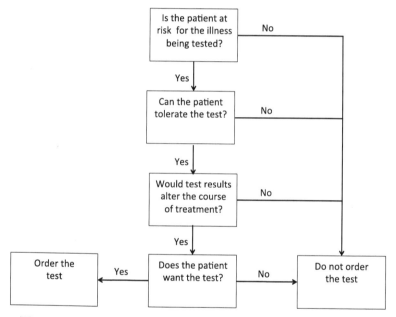

Therefore, informed choice, based on a shared decision-making process that elicits the patient's preferences regarding the diagnostic or treatment decision, should be part of any testing process, whether it be blood, biopsy, or radiological in nature. Reimbursement should be developed to encourage providers and patients to get only appropriate testing that the well-informed patient wants and needs. This process would concurrently discourage overuse of testing, repeat testing, and ordering non-indicated, non-evidence-based, or non-value-added tests.

In summary, as with any medical intervention, testing has both risks and benefits. Patients should be actively informed of both; they should understand how abnormal test results would be addressed, and they should agree to pursue such a course of action. Without that full level of informed, anticipatory understanding of the testing process, testing only adds costs to, and increases the risks of, health care without adding value.

Chapter 6

The Decision

Haley James is a 49-year-old single woman who has suffered from chronic, intermittent back pain of unknown origin for about 20 years. While she attributes the pain to a fall taken while horseback riding, multiple CT and MRI scans have shown no obvious pathology. The pain is so severe that it eventually led to her becoming fully disabled and unable to practice law. Her frustration with ongoing pain has led her to seek care from multiple providers over the years. She has seen a pain specialist who prescribed her methadone and Oxycontin for the pain; she has a neurologist who monitors the pain's progression; she has a general internist who largely manages the consequences of her opiate use, prescribing stool softeners and occasionally addressing severe constipation and compaction issues; and she has a psychiatrist who prescribed antidepressants to help with pain management and to address the depression that is often associated with chronic pain syndromes.

Recently, a new neurosurgical practice opened in town, and Haley, frustrated with having unremitting pain, sought care there. Dr. Jenkins, the neurosurgeon, met her, examined her, and reviewed her extensive chart, x-rays, and other images. "I think we can help you here," he said. "I'd like to operate next week."

"Wow! Hold on," Haley said, somewhat shocked. "A number of physicians have told me that my pain was not amenable to surgical intervention."

"Well, we've made some progress for your condition. I think spinal fusion could help; my patients have had a lot of success with that procedure. I say we get this done sooner rather than later."

"Well, OK, then," Haley said. She was so thankful that she might get some relief from her pain, she eagerly signed up for the surgery. The following Tuesday, Dr. Jenkins saw her in the preoperative room. She was a little groggy, having already received some medications, when she signed the consent form. "Sometimes complications occur," Dr. Jenkins said, "but they're really pretty rare."

In the post-op recovery room, Dr. Jenkins told Haley that things went "very well, no problems." She stayed in the hospital for four days, during which she got a urinary tract infection, and began physical therapy.

Six months after surgery, Haley revisited Dr. Jenkins. "I really don't feel any pain relief," she said. "I'm still on the same medications that I was on before, and the copayments for the surgery cost me over $5,000—that is about four months of my total social security disability income."

"Sometimes it takes longer for things to improve," Dr. Jenkins said. "Be patient."

A year later Haley's pain is unchanged, her medication regimen is the same, and she remains disabled. She is slowly paying off the bill for her hospitalization at a rate of $50 a month. The only difference, she thinks, is that now she has a scar. When she sees her neurologist, he notes a little bit of weakness in her legs, indicating some new nerve compression. "I wish you'd discussed this with me first," he says.

How We Got Here

Historically, patients sought advice and care from physicians, and physicians had largely a paternalistic approach to care. They represented the source of medical knowledge and acted to provide direct guidance as opposed to working with patients to determine which of several options might be the best course of action. While this has changed somewhat over the last 30 years or so, there is still strong evidence that:

1) Where you live determines the intensity of care you get (including the type and number of diagnoses you are given) more than your own health does. In other words, believe it or not, geography is medical destiny: your zip code matters and is a large determinant of what treatment you are likely to receive.

2) Whom you see for medical care (for instance, a surgeon as opposed to an internist) determines what kind of health care you get. Whom you see matters as much as your zip code.

3) Health care providers are at times seemingly more eager to intervene with patients than patients are willing to be intervened with.

4) A number of common and expensive surgical interventions — such as lumbar fusion — appear to have little value in cases like Haley's, and they often lead to ongoing pain and disability.

5) Patients like Haley are often searching for a solution to a set of problems that are difficult at best; sometimes interventions can make things worse. Adequately informing patients like Haley is complicated and confounded by the other treatments and issues surrounding such cases. Workers' compensation, legal issues, chronic pain, the secondary effects of the medical treatments, and the psychological effects of pain all conspire to make such cases even more complex. Treatment options or potential consequences

of different options can be overwhelming and confusing. Cost differences inherent in the treatment options are rarely discussed, and out-of-pocket expenses for surgery and ongoing treatment are rarely, if ever, incorporated into the decision-making process.

Further, with some exceptions, there is little publicly available data on health outcomes or out-of-pocket costs at the provider or health care system level that would allow patients to make informed health care decisions.

What To Do

Often, patients who are experiencing dire circumstances, like Haley, are somewhat desperate; they may be so eager to hear anything positive after enduring a chronic, disabling condition that they might not be able to clearly understand the risks and benefits of particular courses of treatment. This is why objective information about treatment options, potential outcomes and costs associated with each option, and potential downsides of those options should be presented to patients prior to their making a decision. We believe that to reimburse for any services provided, health insurers should demand evidence that such information has been disseminated and that the patient's decision is consistent with his or her values. This is not challenging. Relatively simple measures of decision quality could demonstrate compliance, lead to higher levels of patient satisfaction (because patients' experiences will be consistent with what they anticipated), and reduce health care costs and overutilization of health care resources.

Therefore, completion of shared decision-making and informed choice processes should be a requirement prior to major changes in a course of treatment. However, engaging in such processes can hurt a hospital's bottom line. Because shared decision-making processes generally are not currently funded by insurers, they cost hospitals that use them twice: once in the staff hired to help organize and implement formal shared decision-making processes, and a second time in lost revenues as patients choose less aggressive treatment options after completing a shared decision-making process. Simply requiring evidence that a decision quality score was generated would allow insurers to raise their per-unit reimbursement for more invasive treatment options. Doing so would generate enough savings to pay for the shared decision-making process while still saving money overall, because overall rates of utilization would decrease. Further, insurers would save costs of any complications that might follow the unwarranted or unwanted treatments.

Part of the shared decision-making process should include showing patients who are considering the intervention real-time outcomes of patients who have had similar procedures within the same health care system. These outcomes should include health-related outcomes targeted at what the intervention is intended to address (for instance, pain), complications, and out-of-pocket costs. This data should be collected longitudinally and should include enough baseline information on patient demographics as well as initial symptoms so that the data could be queried to answer the question: How might this procedure impact a patient like me? Further, the shared decision-making process should include similar information from other nearby health care systems so that patients can comparison shop and choose both whether to have an intervention, and if they decide to pursue the intervention, where to get it done. **Figure 6** on the next page shows the shared decision-making process, through which patients receive information on whether and where to obtain a particular course of treatment, payers receive information on decision quality and outcomes, and providers get feedback on their own and other providers' outcomes of care.

Figure 6. The shared decision-making process, through which patients receive information on whether and where to obtain a particular course of treatment, payers receive information on decision quality and outcomes, and providers get feedback on their own and other providers' outcomes of care.

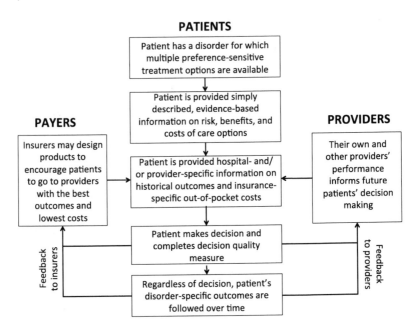

Finally, health care systems should be incentivized to focus more on addressing population health needs than on generating production-based revenues. Changing reimbursement from fee-for-service to capitated methods (and perhaps providing additional financial incentives for demonstrating that shared decision-making processes were used) would help improve patient information, improve patient outcomes, and reduce patient out-of-pocket (and overall health care) costs.

Chapter 7

The Hospital Stay

Ronald Koslowski is a married, 53-year-old man who has diabetes and atherosclerotic disease. He and his wife, Katherine, have been married for 33 years. They have four children (all of whom were out of the house) and three grandchildren, with another on the way. Ron has worked as a pipefitter for the New York State Department of Transportation for 35 years. He and Katherine have excellent health care benefits with very low copayments and coinsurance requirements.

About six months ago, Ron developed chronic stable angina. He was treated with ACE inhibitors, beta-blockers, statins, and nitrates. He continued to have intermittent chest pain, but the pain was not severe and did not really interfere with his work. A coronary angiogram revealed triple vessel disease with 80 percent stenosis of the left main artery. Because of the left main and triple vessel disease, Ron's cardiologist recommended he have coronary artery bypass grafting (CABG) surgery. The cardiologist made the referral, and Ron was scheduled for a triple bypass and showed up at the hospital on the day of surgery.

His was the second scheduled surgery that day, and Ron and Katherine had been told that Ron would head into surgery at 9:30. At about 10:30, one of the residents on the team came in to let Ron and Katherine know that there had been a complication in the previous surgery, and it would be about another hour or so before Ron went into surgery. "We don't do many of these," the resident said. Finally, at 1:00 in the afternoon, Ron was wheeled into surgery. Unfortu-nately, Katherine had gotten so hungry that she'd left to get lunch, so she wasn't there to kiss him good-bye.

Ron woke up in the post-anesthesia care unit (PACU) a little confused. He had multiple tubes in his chest that were draining the wounds, and he had dressings on his right leg where veins had been harvested for the bypass. He stayed in the PACU until his thinking and vital signs improved. He was admitted to his room at 9:30 at night, where an exhausted Katherine greeted him.

Neither Ron nor Katherine got much sleep that night. The monitors kept beeping, and nursing staff woke them every hour to take vital signs. Katherine had to try to sleep in a chair. At about 6 a.m., the team came in as part of their rounds. They asked how Ron felt, and Katherine said he was tired and a little confused. "It was a long surgery, so Ron was on the pump for a little longer than normal," said Dr. Samson, the chief resident.

Over the next couple of days, the drainage tubes were removed, and Ron was up and walking. His pain was well controlled, but he remained a bit confused, Katherine thought. "That's normal," Dr. Samson said. "We'll change his pain meds."

Ron got a urinary tract infection during the stay, but he was able to be discharged after five days in the hospital, on a Saturday. "We've arranged for a home health nurse to come in on Tuesday," the discharge coordinator told Katherine.

"What should he do until then?" Katherine asked.

"Well, just do your best," the discharge coordinator said.

Thankfully, two of Ron's children lived nearby, and they were available to help Katherine manage Ron's care and to help Ron get around for the next few days. The home health nurse came on Tuesday afternoon and interviewed Ron and Katherine; Katherine was still worried that Ron was a little confused. "That'll probably get better with time," the nurse said.

After a couple more weeks, Ron returned to work. Ron's supervisor,

Jim, called Katherine at noon on Ron's first day back. "Are you sure he's ready to come back?" Jim asked. "He doesn't really seem all 'there.'"

"The doctors said he could go back three weeks after the surgery, and it's been three weeks," Katherine answered.

"Has he been back to the doctors?"

"No...he's scheduled to see them in another couple of weeks."

At the return visit, Katherine again noted that Ron seemed a bit confused. "Also, he just doesn't seem to have much energy," she said. Ron was pretty passive during the visit.

"Sometimes patients get depressed after heart surgery. I'll put him on Prozac and he should see a psychiatrist," the doctor said. "His scars look great, though. And he's not had any chest pain, so that's a good thing."

Katherine went with Ron to his psychiatric appointment and described the changes that had occurred since the surgery: Ron seemed to get easily confused, he seemed a bit lethargic, and since the Prozac was started, he wasn't interested in sex at all. Dr. Viceroy, the psychiatrist, had completed a fellowship in health services research. He told Katherine that one common side effect of Prozac is sexual dysfunction, and that different medications could be used if Ron was depressed, which was, indeed, a common occurrence after CABG.

"How did you choose the hospital where Ron got his surgery?" Dr. Viceroy asked.

"We just went where the cardiologist told us to go," Katherine answered.

Ron continued to see Dr. Viceroy, who asked that some psychological testing be completed. The testing showed some mild neurological deficits that were likely attributable to a longer-than-expected time on the heart pump during surgery. Ron's depression got better with a different medication that did not have negative sexual side effects, and his neurological deficits seemed to slowly improve.

"That's too bad," Dr. Viceroy told the psychologist while reviewing the testing results. "The hospital that Ron went to has had

the worse risk-adjusted CABG outcomes of any hospital in New York for the past 10 years—New York's Statewide Planning and Research Cooperative System has been publicly reporting results for every CABG center in New York for more than 30 years. I just can't believe that data was not part of the decision-making process for Ron and Katherine."

How We Got Here

For many years, health care has been largely organized around providers. Certainly, patients needed access to providers to get care, and they needed to be seen by providers to have tests, referrals, and procedures arranged. But little emphasis has been placed on patient needs; patients were generally peripheral to the care-delivery process. An air of paternalism permeated health care delivery; patients saw providers at the providers' convenience; they obtained care wherever providers had referral networks; and they largely followed providers' direction, relatively passively.

In part, this was a cultural phenomenon. In the first three-quarters of the twentieth century, physicians were highly regarded and respected, and the country, as a whole, was more accepting of paternalistic relationships, whether the source of paternalism was the authority of government, religious bodies, or employers. However, as has been noted, the methods of health care delivery and reimbursement were largely established in the United States between World War II and the early 1970s, during which time employer-based insurance for members of the labor force and government-based insurance for retirees and those unable to work were established.

Since the 1970s there has been a cultural shift, with a rise of independent thinking and a substantial increase in tolerance for different opinions. These shifts were undoubtedly fostered by a response to the Vietnam War, the civil rights movement, the feminist movement, and other social movements. Regardless of the source, the reality is that paternalism as a social construct has fallen to the wayside, and the ready availability of information on the Internet is likely to keep it there.

But there is a considerable amount of misinformation on the Internet, and it is difficult to determine what medical information is accurate and useful. Unfortunately, studies have shown that the types of information that have been provided by independent agencies, such as New York's Department of Health, are rarely used by patients in determining where to get care. For instance, New York's Statewide Planning and Research Cooperative System has provided physician- and hospital-specific information on risk-adjusted mortality and morbidity rates for all New York hospitals (except for VA or Department of Defense hospitals) that provide CABG or percutaneous coronary interventions since the late 1970s. While there is evidence that providers have changed practice — some low performers either went out of business or moved to a different state — and that such changes have improved outcomes, there is still substantial variation in risk-adjusted rates. Some years, one hospital will have rates that are two or three times higher than others. While the hospitals do not tend to make this information available, the Department of Health does. Unfortunately, not all states provide these services. And only rarely do New York residents who are considering CABG surgery use this information.

In a similar vein, much research has identified a "volume-outcomes" relationship between health outcomes and the number of times a particular procedure is performed each year by a provider or within a hospital. The relationship makes sense; practice makes perfect. And while understanding that the measure is imperfect, a group of large employers called the Leapfrog Group has tried to integrate adherence to minimum volume standards (for instance, a minimum of 450 CABG surgeries per year and a minimum of 11 pancreatic resections per year) into hospital referral practices.

Unfortunately, insurers have not tended to use this type of information — anticipated outcomes that are based on either historic mortality rates or procedure volumes — in their benefits design. In part because of concerns about backlash from consumers about provider or hospital choice, insurers have been reluctant to use benefits design to "steer" the patients they insure to lower mortality hospitals.

While the vignette in this chapter outlines the lack of evidence-based referral practices, it demonstrates that there continues to be a problem implementing what is known to work in a timely manner. For some time a strong association between depression and recent CABG has been established; therefore, it should be common practice for providers to seek to identify and treat symptoms of depression in patients who have recently had CABG surgery. While like all medications, antidepressants certainly do have side effects that should be explained to patients as part of the informed consent process, in many cases antidepressants should be preemptively prescribed for patients undergoing CABG surgery, as taking these medications improves outcomes.

Clearly, Ron's hospitalization seems to have been disjointed and lacked much evidence of care coordination, solid follow-up care, explanation of side effects or potential complications, or good management of care transitions. Intriguingly, virtually all parties involved in Ron's care would have benefited had care options, side effects, and transitions been clearly explained: Ron and Katherine would have been better informed and might have chosen a different hospital that might have had better outcomes; the providers would have provided more thorough informed consent and had less of a liability problem; and the insurer might have incurred lower health care costs by directing

Ron's care to a high-volume, high-value provider.

What To Do

This case demonstrates tremendous opportunities for using shared decision-making or informed-choice processes, including taking advantage of the availability of transparent outcomes and cost data in that shared decision-making process, using benefits design to steer patients toward high-value providers, and exploiting market pressures to improve health care value.

First, it should be self-evident that patient referrals should not be based only on referral networks. Patients should be provided information on different treatment options, different places where they might obtain the care they choose, the risk-adjusted outcomes of those different places, and importantly, the short-term and estimated long-term out-of-pocket costs that any of their treatment options will involve.

Earlier, we contended that a simple measure of "decision quality" be incorporated into how health care value is calculated; further, we think that insurers should require that decision quality be measured for major medical decisions before they reimburse for those procedures. Such a measure would ensure that providers review patients' treatment options, provide documentation that patients have participated in an "informed choice" process, and that patients are at the center of the decision-making process.

In addition, insurers might use benefits design to steer patients toward higher-value care providers. For instance, while retaining choice, patients might be incentivized to choose high-value care through new benefits structures: patients might have lower out-of-pocket costs or copayments if they choose to use hospitals with excellent risk-adjusted outcomes over hospitals with poorer outcomes. This might benefit all parties. Patients like Ron might have experienced lower out-of-pocket costs if he had chosen a hospital with better outcomes and higher volumes. Insurers might have paid less for the episode of care (and for overall health care services) at a hospital that had demonstrated higher-quality, better-outcomes care. Finally, the providers might have benefited from increased volumes generated as a result of more patients improving the health care team's experience and outcomes and driving down the hospital's costs per unit, making them more profitable.

Figure 7 shows what might happen if insurers used benefit design to "steer" patients to higher-quality care (in this case, using risk-adjusted mortality rates as the indicator of quality).

Figure 7. An example of using benefits design to "steer" patients to higher-quality care.

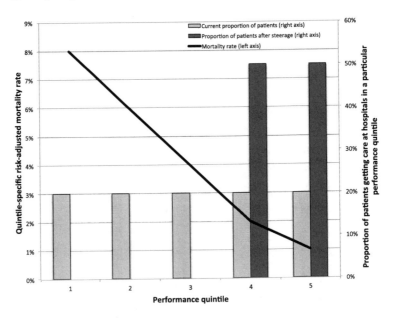

In the example, each performance quintile has a different risk-adjusted mortality rate, declining from 8 percent in the worst performing quintile to 1 percent in the best performing quintile. Without steerage, one-fifth of the population obtains care in each quintile, and the average mortality rate that the population could expect is 4.2 percent. But if insurers provided incentives that encouraged patients to obtain care from providers in the best two performance quintiles, the average mortality rate that the population could expect drops by almost two-thirds, to 1.5 percent. While some might be concerned that patients would have fewer hospitals from which to choose, the benefits could be designed to allow patients to choose a lower performance care setting, but without the reduced copayment.

While health care value is traditionally defined as quality and outcomes divided by costs, patients should be involved in determining what is high quality. For instance, the lack of basic hotel services that required Katherine to try to sleep on a chair, the lack of prompt follow-up (with either the home health nurse or the physician), and the apparent lack of orientation of Ron and Katherine to the health care delivery process are all important to patients and should be measured and reported on. Just as one might look at a Consumer Reports–type of assessment of quality before buying a car, there are multiple aspects of care that patients might reasonably value differently. While some car purchasers may think that car repair records are the most important aspect of quality, others may put more emphasis on better gas mileage. Transparently providing information on a variety of aspects of health care quality that patients value would allow them to make informed health care decisions and align those decisions with their own health care values.

In our view, a combination of out-of-pocket cost estimates, quality, and outcome measures should be readily available and transparently presented so that a patient can answer the question: How might this intervention impact a patient like me? Such data should be available to patients, insurers, and other providers.

The integration of this data into the decision-making process is paramount to bending the cost curve; by letting patients sit in the driver's seat and make informed decisions, by encouraging them to get only the care they want and need, and by designing benefits that use behavior economics techniques that encourage patients to choose the highest-value care, health care costs should decline and health care quality and outcomes should improve. If widespread, such information would drive patients to use higher-value care, concentrate care among the highest-value providers, and improve the national value of delivered health care by driving down costs and improving health outcomes.

Chapter 8

The Postoperative, Post-Acute- Care Period

Victor Cheever is an active and healthy 73-year-old man who has had long-standing knee osteoarthritis dating all the way back to a football injury in high school. Victor enjoys walking and hiking, but his knee pain was getting too extreme for him to enjoy these activities as much as he would have liked. He lives with Jenny, his wife of 52 years, in northern New Hampshire, "close enough to the Canadian border to escape there, if they institute an income tax here," he liked to joke, as New Hampshire has no state income tax. Where he lives allows him to experience wilderness and to hike regularly in the White Mountains, but he is a distance from inpatient health care services. To address the increasing knee pain, he had tried analgesic medications, physical therapy steroid injections, and even Synvisc—an artificial knee joint lubricant—all without long-lasting pain relief.

"Sometimes, when there is trauma involved, the osteoarthritis is more resistant to the conservative treatments. Perhaps it's time to consider knee replacement surgery," said Dr. Fredericks, the orthopedic surgeon. Dr. Fredericks arranged for Victor to go to the shared decision-making center, where he went through an "informed choice" process with his wife prior to choosing knee replacement surgery.

Victor made the three-hour trip to the hospital with his wife the evening before surgery; they stayed in a local hotel to make sure they made it to the pre-op appointment in the morning in plenty of time. The surgery went off without a hitch, and Victor was discharged to a rehabilitation hospital three days after the operation. By then Jenny was getting tired—the bed in the hospital room was not comfortable for her, and she didn't want to stay in the hotel.

"Does he really need to go to a rehab hospital?" Jenny asked.

"That's our protocol here," the physical therapist responded.

"But couldn't I take him home and get home care? They have it; I checked."

"Well, we really prefer to send the patients to rehabilitation hospitals. They're part of our system, and we feel that provides better integrated care for our patients."

So Victor was transferred by ambulance to the rehabilitation hospital where he stayed and received physical therapy for a week. After a couple of nights there, Jenny drove home and waited for a daily call that updated her on Victor's progress. She returned at the end of the week to pick Victor up. He was walking and stable and told her that the pain was gone. "I can't wait to get back on the trails," he told her.

A week after that, and then the week after, Jenny and Victor drove down for follow-up visits at the hospital. Each of the visits lasted perhaps 10 minutes after the doctor finally arrived (one time he was 45 minutes late for the appointment). During the visits Dr. Fredericks asked how he was, whether there was any pain, and looked at the suture line.

About two months after the operation, Jenny opened the bill for the hospitalization. She was shocked that the cost was more than $40,000, but she was relieved that, because of the Medigap policy they had, their out-of-pocket costs were very modest. Then, about four days later, another bill for $18,000 arrived from the rehabilitation hospital. A week after that, the bill for the physician component of the hospital stay arrived—about $8,000 for the surgeon, the *anesthesiologist, and the outpatient visits. Finally, the bill for the ambulance service was about $1,000.*

Jenny became interested in different care patterns for knee replacement surgery, and after completing an Internet search, she found 17 hospitals in the region that did knee replacement surgery and that described the care process. About one-third appeared to have a general practice of discharging patients to home with home health follow-up and local physical therapy; about one-third appeared to discharge patients to skilled nursing facilities; and about one-third appeared to discharge patients to rehabilitation hospitals. She seemed to find a pattern: when hospitals discharged patients to rehabilitation hospitals, both the hospital where the surgery was done and the rehabilitation hospital were frequently owned by the same health care system.

Jenny and Victor are pleased with the results of the surgery, but they wonder whether health care delivery might be more consistent across the different hospitals that provided essentially the same services. To them, after discharge it seemed that almost all of the health care services provided could have been done by phone.

"I know we didn't have to pay for the rehabilitation and extra services," Victor says. "But Medicare is going bankrupt, and I hate to have contributed to that, even unwittingly."

How We Got Here

Hospital revenues were pinched by the transition from a cost-plus formula to the diagnosis related group (DRG) reimbursement mechanism that now defines a hybrid type of fee-for-service payment system; while hospitals are indeed reimbursed for the total hospitalization on a DRG basis, they were previously reimbursed for each service provided during the hospitalization. So, in essence, hospitalizations were "bundled" in the early 1980s into DRGs.

Hospitals responded to this change in reimbursement methodology by shortening stays and outsourcing some services. One way in which hospitals outsourced services was to disaggregate rehabilitative services from acute hospitalization services; without transfer to a different facility, any rehabilitative services would be considered part of the acute hospitalization. Therefore, to maximize system-wide revenue, hospitals affiliated with and created networks with rehabilitation hospitals and skilled nursing facilities. In that way the hospital could obtain full DRG reimbursement for the inpatient admission and transfer the patient to a skilled nursing facility or a rehabilitation hospital for rehabilitation. That second rehabilitation hospitalization would be billed and reimbursed separately.

To further complicate things, hospital services and physician services are frequently billed separately, so individuals like Victor and Jenny might receive multiple bills for a single hospitalization—or, as in this case, two hospitalizations, with the second being in the rehabilitation setting. These multiple bills seem to obfuscate costs and confuse patients. Such billing can also accelerate health care spending, as part of Victor's care was likely optional and added little if any to his outcome, but added a lot to the overall cost of his care.

What To Do

While bundling all services—including outpatient, preadmission, hospitalization, and follow-up care (including that received in rehabilitation hospitals, skilled nursing facilities, or through home health care)—for a 30-day episode of care might appear to be a good initial solution, it, too, has potential downfalls. First, bundling would certainly reduce hospitals' use of unnecessary care as well as efforts to admit patients who otherwise might not need care in an effort to fill owned rehabilitation hospitals and skilled nursing facilities. And bundling of physician services—and even pharmaceutical costs—into the overall episode of care would provide incentives to reduce unnecessary consultation and high-cost, nongeneric medication use.

However, as happened when hospital care was bundled into DRGs, hospitals might respond to efforts to bundle costs of episodes of care by simply increasing volumes of care provided. There is considerable evidence that physicians continue to determine rates of admission for care—for elective surgeries such as knee replacement surgery or coronary artery bypass grafting, they can be more persuasive or simply lower the threshold for treatment, frequently without even being aware they are doing so. So episode-based bundling without a responsibility for management of overall population rates of admissions will have the same effects as hospitalization bundling did under DRGs: the lengths of stay would decrease, and some services would be reduced, but overall volumes would increase, considerably, and cost savings generated by the bundling process would be more than offset by increased volumes of care.

Therefore, system-specific information on costs and outcomes of care should be provided to encourage care improvement. **Figure 8** on the next page provides an example of how the composition and amount of post-acute-care costs in the 30 days following discharge might vary across health care systems for a particular admission type. It is evident that the total costs of post-acute-care vary from about $2,000 to almost $10,000. Further, health care systems' use of physician care, home health care, and rehabilitation care vary considerably.

Such data should be collected and presented to different health care systems to allow them to identify best practices in post-acute-care management.

Further, although the vignette demonstrated the use of a shared decision-making process regarding whether or not to get knee replacement surgery, that decision-making process failed to provide transparency regarding out-of-pocket costs, care alternatives, and the impact of different care pathways on

Figure 8. An example of how the composition and amount of post-acute-care costs in the thirty days following discharge might vary across health-care systems for a particular admission type.

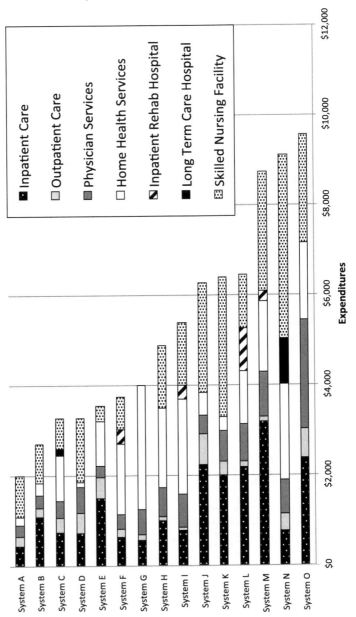

out-of-pocket costs. Indeed, comparisons of alternatives in the general market or region—such as the one Jenny did herself, after the fact—might have helped Victor make an even better decision regarding when, where, and what type of care he wanted to receive. Information like that shown in **Figure 8** might have helped Victor anticipate costs of care as well as the post-acute-care process.

The keys to improving the efficiency and value created by post-acute-care are to do the following: align incentives so that health care systems eradicate waste; improve transparency of data on costs, outcomes, and care-process choices; and have a laser-like focus on determining and providing what patients want and need—and only that.

Chapter 9

The Bill

A young couple, Joe and Lucinda Ramirez, were expecting their first child. They were healthy and happy and eagerly anticipating their first addition to the family. As a birthday surprise for Lucinda, Joe had spent several weekends refurbishing a closet in their small house to serve as a nursery, one painted in light blue with clouds painted across the walls and ceiling. "I want him to feel like he's flying," Joe told Lucinda when he finally showed her the room.

About three months prior to the due date, Lucinda fainted at home and began having seizures. Joe called 9-1-1, and an ambulance came and took her to the nearest hospital, which was not the one where Lucinda had received her prenatal care. In the emergency room, Lucinda regained consciousness. She and a terrified Joe were told that Lucinda had eclampsia and that she still had very high blood pressure. The emergency room physician said Lucinda was not responding well to typical anti-eclampsia medications and recommended that an emergency cesarean section be performed, for Lucinda's sake and for the sake of the baby. A C-section was performed, and a very tiny Juan was born and immediately placed in the neonatal ICU.

Lucinda stayed in the hospital for four days, recovering from her C-section; Joe took off work to be with Lucinda and Juan. Juan had a variety of complications associated with being born prematurely. He was not able to breastfeed and therefore required total intravenous nutrition. When Lucinda and Joe came to visit him, they thought

Juan looked like a porcupine, with needles and tubes sticking out of him. When he was 14 days old, Juan developed bleeding within his brain and began having seizures, a not-uncommon occurrence in premature births. "This means that he's lost some brain tissue," Dr. Lester, the neurosurgeon, told them. "Many times children can recover, but often there is lasting brain damage."

Juan developed hydrocephalus from the hemorrhage, and consultations were obtained from occupational and physical therapy, as well as child neurology. "The key is early intervention," each of the consultants said. A shunt was implanted that moved the excess cerebrospinal fluid into Juan's abdomen; Joe and Lucinda could see a small tube protruding under Juan's thin skin that wandered from his head, down his neck, along his sternum, and into his abdomen.

While Lucinda and Joe spent as much time as they could at the hospital, they both had jobs, and they were running out of cash. One morning at 3:25 a.m., they received a call. "Little Juan died," Nurse Engles told them. "I'm really sorry." Juan had died when he was 27 days old.

They had a ceremony for Juan and buried him in a family plot, next to Joe's grandfather. The little nursery seemed a colder and darker place than it had been before. Still, Joe spent time there, thinking about the life that little Juan might have had.

The day after the funeral, Joe received a bill for the ambulance service for Lucinda. About three days later, he received a bill for the emergency room physician services. The day after that, he received a bill for the C-section and Lucinda's hospital stay. And four weeks after Juan's funeral service, Joe received a bill for Juan's 27-day hospital stay in the ICU and surgical interventions for $1,267,914. A week after that, he received additional charges for physician services for Juan's neonatologist, neurosurgeon, and anesthesiologist, and bills for the physical therapist, occupational therapist, and neurologist consults.

In total, the bills exceeded $1.5 million; they were presented across about 200 pages of paper. Some of the bills provided incredible *detail—for instance, the hospital bill included a daily breakdown of the types of hospital services provided. Some were much less specific, such as the single item for the neurosurgical placement of the shunt. Every bill showed the original charge, the charge to the insurance company, the amount that the insurance company paid, and in bold letters, the amount that Joe and Lucinda "saved" by virtue of their insurance company's negotiating skills. The remainder—the amount that Joe and Lucinda owed the hospital and the various providers in copayments, coinsurance, and deductibles—amounted to $73,216.*

Joe had no idea how he was supposed to pay for this. He and Lucinda had a combined income of about $75,000 a year and at ages 27 and 29, very little savings. "I guess we'll have to declare bankruptcy," Joe thought, after speaking to the hospital's financial adviser.

How We Got Here

As discussed earlier, health care insurance became widely available as a result of wage freezes during World War II, when companies provided such insurance to attract workers when only a paucity of them existed. Broadly, two types of insurance were available: insurance for hospital stays and insurance for physician services. This system of separating insurance for hospital care and physician was cemented in the establishment of Medicare, which provided hospital care reimbursement through Part A and physician care and other health care services reimbursement through Part B.

So, historically, different types of care generated different bills; further, different companies (for instance, ambulance care services and physician practices) might request Part B equivalent reimbursement separately, so bills that a patient might feel were related to the same general service might come from separate entities at different times. This tends to confuse patients, who might believe that one bill simply covered all the services provided during an episode of care.

And hospital bills are confusing for other reasons as well. As shown in the vignette in this chapter, some bills provide extensive detail—perhaps more than is needed—while some provide cursory explanations of charges. Patients who compare hospital bills across different type of service providers might be confused because "facility fees" might be captured on one bill, but bills for the professional services rendered during the same event might be captured on an entirely different bill.

Another confusing aspect of health care bills are the "discounts" that insurers show on the bill. Insurers like to demonstrate to their clients that they have "saved" them money. Therefore, insurers demand steep discounts when negotiating with hospitals and providers for final reimbursement. To be able to provide those discounts, these providers simply ratchet up their "rack rates" (akin to a list price, the rack rate is the rate from which discounts are taken). They actually calculate the rack rate based on the anticipated payer-mix that they will experience (the proportion of their patients who are insured by different insurances, such as Medicare and Medicaid, which tend to reimburse at lower rates and do not negotiate rates). They then set rack rates at a level that allows a hefty discount for commercial insurers (so they can tell their beneficiaries that they saved them money). Because virtually no person will ever pay the rack rate (even self-pay patients can easily negotiate steep discounts from these), the rack rate is a fiction that distorts pricing information; there is no relationship between costs and rack rates, and rack rates are not related to actual reimbursements. Therefore, almost no information is conveyed to markets from rack rates.

However, rack rates command quite a bit of attention when they are presented, generally in sensationalistic news magazines, and even in research articles. Unfortunately, while the demonstration of these rates seeks to show wide variation in health care expenses and some extraordinary costs of care, because the rack rates do not reflect the amounts that either patients or insurers pay, such reports are truly misleading.

Nonetheless, health care bills can accelerate quickly, as is shown in this case. And because there are often no caps on medical expenses for a hospital stay, medical expenses continue to be the most frequent cause of bankruptcy in America today.

What To Do

Several steps could be taken to improve billing practices. First, additional "bundling" of services — for instance, including the costs of all services associated with an episode of care, including hospital costs, physician costs, ancillary service costs, and all associated fees — can help make billing simpler and can curtail the kind of excesses that generate news stories (like $10 aspirin pills). In particular, if such charges were presented in advance as a prospective payment amount, similar to DRGs, this would help payers and patients understand anticipated costs.

Further, because patients are interested in the out-of-pocket expenses they might incur during a course of treatment, those costs should be presented as well. While these might differ according to insurance status, revealing them would help patients make more informed decisions around where to obtain care — they could see what copayments, coinsurance, and deductibles for particular courses of action would cost them and thereby make more informed treatment decisions.

Instead of a confusing bill that itemizes each care component and applies seemingly random discounts to charges, one could imagine a simple bill that provided the negotiated overall costs of an episode of care (**Figure 9** on the following page). Integrated into the bill might be the transparent incentive that was provided if a patient chose a high-performance provider.

Figure 9. An example of what a current and future bill for an admission for hip replacement surgery might look like.

Current

Date	Item	Charge	Insurance reduction	You owe
7/4/15	Preoperative anesthetic	$1,364.92	$505.02	$859.90
7/4/15	Postoperative anesthetic	$842.96	$362.47	$480.49
7/4/15	Nursing care in preoperative waiting	$967.40	$561.09	$406.31
7/4/15	Nursing care in post-operative recovery	$1,473.87	$854.84	$619.03
7/4/15	Transportation services	$78.34	$28.20	$50.14
7/4/15	Operating room charge	$2,688.44	$940.95	$1,747.49
7/4/15	Implant	$5,922.88	$2,487.61	$3,435.27
7/4/15	Food services	$23.45	$14.07	$9.38
7/4/15	Postoperative ibuprofen (400 mg)	$5.66	$3.40	$2.26
7/4/15	Postoperative ibuprofen (400 mg)	$5.66	$3.40	$2.26
7/4/15	Postoperative ibuprofen (400 mg)	$7.66	$3.40	$2.26
	Page 1 of 9			$7,614.79

Future

7/4–8/9/15	Admission for hip replacement and 30-day follow-up care	$16,592.00	$14,932.80	$1,659.20
	Reduction in care costs because you chose a high-performance system		$1,659.20	$0.00

Finally, patients should be protected from bankruptcy that results from medical misfortune. This can be accomplished in several ways. First, insurers could provide a collaborative reinsurance pool that they can incorporate into their premium pricing. Spread across an entire insured population, such costs would be minimal at the patient level. Second, government policies that would preclude bankruptcy from medical misfortune could be enacted. Just as the federal government can bail out large banks or auto manufacturers, it could effectively use tax resources to preclude the possibility that individuals would go bankrupt as a result of receiving needed medical care.

Certainly, hospitals and health-care providers could obtain reinsurance to cover the costs of care that exceed a certain amount. This, too, could prevent individuals from needing to declare bankruptcy in order to eradicate excessive debt related to medical misfortune; further, it would ensure that hospitals and health-care providers do not unfairly bear the brunt of unpaid care. The additional per-service costs of the necessary reinsurance would be minimal.

Chapter 10

The Management
of Chronic Disease

Alex Howell is the 44-year-old single mother of James, a seven-year-old boy with chronic asthma. Alex has three part-time jobs, none of which provide health care insurance. She makes too much money to qualify for Medicaid, and the insurance policies afforded by the ACA insurance exchange are too expensive for her. She tried to obtain additional services for single mothers through the state, but the paperwork was complex and difficult for her to complete. One social worker suggested that Alex try to pursue disability status, but Alex, though she has chronic and somewhat painful rheumatoid arthritis, says she does not want to "be a burden" on the system. She works hard and is responsible and well liked by her bosses; however, James has had several asthma attacks that landed him in the hospital and required her to miss work unexpectedly. Alex has lost three part-time jobs in the past two years because of these hospitalizations. Therefore, she generally paid for health care expenses out of pocket.

Alex was at work when James's after-school care provider called her on a Friday afternoon. James was showing classic symptoms of an impending asthma attack; there was a cold going around, and James was pretty susceptible to colds. Usually, antibiotics and a nebulizer could help stave off the attack. But Alex was at work until five, and her primary care physician's office closed then. She called the primary care physician's office, but they had only seen James once (the old primary care physician had left), and they did not want to prescribe anything without seeing him first.

"But this has worked every time for the last few years," Alex said. "He gets really sick without getting the antibiotics and nebulizer."

"There's an epidemic of antibiotic overuse in America, and we're committed to help try to stop that," the receptionist responded. "In fact, one of our performance measures is focused on reducing antibiotic use in pediatric patients."

"What should I do?" Alex asked.

"You can go to the ER. They can evaluate James and prescribe antibiotics if that's appropriate."

Alex picked up James at five thirty; his asthma was worse, and he was wheezing. She had him try a couple of puffs on his inhaler, but that did not relieve his symptoms for long. She drove James to the emergency room, where they waited for four hours to be seen. During that time James's breathing got more strained. By the time he was seen, he was audibly wheezing and was having some intercostal retractions (retractions of the chest muscles).

"We can give him a nebulizer and some antibiotics," said Dr. Jenson, the ER pediatrician. "We'd like to watch him for a while."

At four thirty in the morning, James was released from the ER; his breathing was no longer labored, and the nebulizer had worked. He had received one dose of antibiotics and had had an additional prescription for a full course of antibiotics to be taken over the next week called in to a pharmacy.

Alex needed to get to work at six thirty, and James's day care started at six fifteen. They were both exhausted, but Alex got James some cereal, she got herself a cup of coffee, and she began to get them ready at five thirty. Fortunately, the day-care provider had some experience with asthma and was fine with James needing to take antibiotics. "Poor kid," she said, when Alex was describing their night.

Three weeks later Alex got a bill for $2,200 for the emergency room visit.

How We Got Here

The U.S. health care system was largely designed around acute-care management for good reason; as a more formal health care system was developing in the early 1900s, there was simply not much chronic disease. People did not survive long enough to get chronic diseases, or at least they were not recognized as such. Primarily, the goal was to help patients survive an acute disorder.

One of the population consequences of the U.S. health care system's ability to better manage acute disorders is that large numbers of people who survive have chronic conditions. For instance, survivors of heart attacks have angina or congestive heart failure; survivors of strokes develop organic personality disorders; and survivors of different kinds of cancers develop chronic disorders associated with relapse prevention. The management of chronic diseases requires different skill sets than does management of acute disorders. While preventive and public health goals include taking preventive measures to help patients avoid the underlying physiologic changes that lead to acute disorders, chronic disease management attempts to prevent worsening of the underlying disorder, once it has been established.

The vignette at the beginning of this chapter demonstrates that earlier intervention and better chronic-care management can improve patient care, improve outcomes, and reduce resource consumption.

The vignette also demonstrates the importance of easy access to care when acute exacerbations occur within chronic disease conditions. Importantly, allowing patients to use more self-management techniques — including even determining the course of care and the required interventions — would seemingly result in better outcomes at lower costs. In this case, Alex was very familiar with James's chronic condition and how to prevent asthma attacks; indeed, she "prescribes" exactly what the emergency room doctor later prescribed. Informed by experience, her approach to disease management would have saved thousands of dollars and provided earlier symptom relief for James. However, her access to primary care was restricted, and as the primary care providers acted as gateway managers to what had been an effective course of treatment, the provision of that treatment was compromised.

Further, the vignette demonstrates that concerns about internal performance measures might preclude appropriate use of antibiotics. While performance management systems help drive higher-value care, their mostly blind application has the potential to undermine care for individual patients. As previously discussed, some health care systems' performances are determined, in part, by the degree to which they perform colonoscopies in patients who are aged 50 and older. But some patients might not warrant such preventive care; for instance, patients who are very ill, patients who prefer not to have the screening procedure, and patients whose colons have been removed.

What To Do

Clearly, the vignette articulates the need for broad insurance coverage for patients. Insurance coverage improves access to care, and earlier access to care can improve health care outcomes. Despite the fact that Alex had some access to care, she made too much money to qualify for one form of health insurance and too little to afford another.

Intriguingly, from a systems standpoint, had Alex had insurance coverage, everyone in the case might have been better off. Clearly James would have been better off—he would have perhaps had better access to preventive health care services. Alex would have had peace of mind, and in the event she needed emergency room services, the bill might have not been so high. And the emergency room would have been better reimbursed had Alex had insurance coverage; as it stands, the emergency room is not likely to be paid for the services rendered there.

Many studies have shown that use of technology, chronic-care pathways, self-management tools, and improved care access improve chronic-care outcomes. Unfortunately, insurers may not reimburse many of these services; therefore, it is incumbent on health care systems to provide such reimbursed care. Ironically, provision for such services frequently generates a loss of revenues for the health care system that provides them, as provision for acute-care services tends to reimburse at higher rates than preventive care services do. An example of a current and future way of providing chronic-care treatment is shown in **Figure 10** on the next page.

Incentives to engage patients in health maintenance, to structure their benefits to improve their use of preventive and ongoing monitoring services, and to encourage the use of self-management tools designed to avoid use of acute-care services would reduce insurance costs and improve patient-care outcomes. Moreover, encouraging patients to access such care from a distance—through telephone, e-mail, or mobile applications—would improve care access, reduce health care costs, and improve health care providers' efficiency. We believe there is the potential for out-of-hospital chronic-disease management to save 30 percent of current health care costs. The new technologies needed for such care management processes will accelerate the industrial revolution in health care over the next five to 10 years.

Figure 10. Current and future methods for providing chronic-care management.

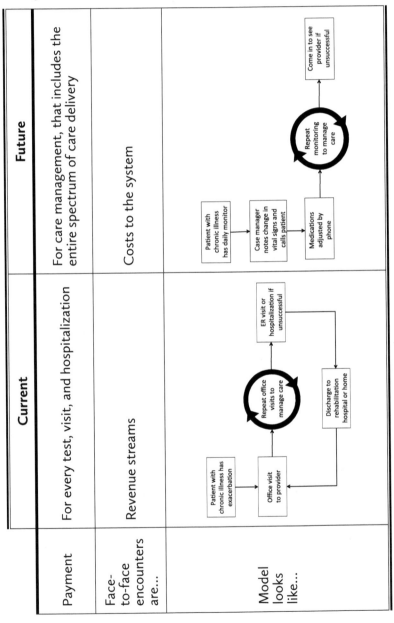

Chapter 11

The Management of Dying

Stephanie Watson was an elderly, widowed woman with multiple medical conditions who lived in a nursing home. One of her comorbidities was Alzheimer's disease that had been progressively worsening. Stephanie had an advanced directive that she completed when in the earlier stages of Alzheimer's; the advanced directive indicated her desire not to die in the hospital or to receive intensive treatment should she be on the cusp of death. Her son, Richard, lived several states away and could visit only irregularly; on his last visit, Stephanie only vaguely seemed to recognize him.

On a Saturday morning, Stephanie developed pneumonia; the doctor on call at the nursing home saw her, noted some increased confusion and difficulty breathing, and sent her to the emergency room. In the ER she was evaluated, diagnosed with pneumonia, and admitted to the hospital. During the hospital stay, Stephanie was disoriented and confused. Her mild congestive heart failure worsened, and she became sluggish and confused and developed severe heart failure.

Unfortunately, the hospital did not have a copy of her advanced directive, and they could not reach Richard or her attending physician, so they proceeded with acute-care management. Stephanie's course worsened, and she was eventually admitted to the ICU, where she was put on intravenous nutrition and fluids.

On Monday the hospital was finally able to reach Richard, who immediately drove to the hospital and brought a copy of the advanced directive. He was upset to see his mother in an ICU, unresponsive, having difficulty breathing, and covered with medical equipment.

"This isn't what she wanted at all," he said. "Why didn't you all have the advance directive?"

The hospital risk manager explained that because of privacy concerns (the Health Insurance Portability and Accountability Act provides strict guidelines about the sharing of health information, violations of which can result in substantial penalties to health-care providers), the hospital was unable to obtain the advance directive from the nursing home. "We feel ethically obliged to offer aggressive treatment when there is no evidence of an advance directive. Now that we have one, we can get an ethics consultation if you'd like to remove treatment."

An ethics consultation was obtained, the advance directive was reviewed, and Richard was interviewed. The team concurred that Ms. Watson would not have wanted to endure the treatment to which she had been subjected. She was discharged from the ICU to the floor, the intravenous nutrition and fluids were withdrawn, and she died three days later.

About six weeks after the funeral, Richard received a bill for the week-long hospital stay that exceeded $50,000; the out-of-pocket costs that were not covered by insurance and would be owed by his mother's estate amounted to $11,368.

Richard cried.

How We Got Here

Historically, health care has had almost a laser-like focus on acute-care management. Only recently has chronic-disease management and considerations of end-of-life care come into the forefront of health-care delivery. But this focus on acute care, combined with a sense that everything that is wrong should be addressed and fixed, as well as a fear of legal retribution if such a course of action were not taken, have all conspired to drive overuse of health care and waste of health-care resources, which are most apparent at end-of-life care.

In addition, the lack of integration of acute-care services (such as hospitals and emergency rooms) with chronic-care services (such as nursing homes and home health care) has exacerbated communication problems across providers. Even if each of these systems of care had its own electronic health records, those systems have been designed as stand-alone systems that do not communicate with one another. These systems have been largely designed around billing and tend to serve the needs of the health-care provider; they have not been designed around patient-centered clinical care management.

Fears of legal action have distorted health-care services delivery from two perspectives. First, while entities are exceedingly rarely sued because they did too much, they are much more commonly sued if experts suggest they did too little. In this case, because the hospital was unable to contact a relative and the patient was incompetent to make medical decisions, the legal environment compelled the staff to provide extensive health-care services, even if they might have thought such treatment was futile. Second, concerns about legal ramifications of not protecting personal health information may lead to costly delays in communicating with critical providers.

What to Do

This vignette demonstrates the need to identify patients at risk for becoming very ill very quickly, to develop plans for what course of action to take should that occur and to widely communicate that plan. While integration of electronic health records across the different provider types would help with this communication, better yet would be to design health records that are portable, patient centered, comprehensive, and that travel with the patient. Then plans would be readily available to treatment providers at any time.

Although the vignette focused on the excesses of care in the hospital setting, a critical error was made in the initial decision to send Ms. Watson to the hospital for treatment. Here again, anticipation of rapid worsening of her physical condition might have helped determine a better course of action. Palliative care for patients with terminal diseases such as Alzheimer's disease can be tailored to home or nursing home settings. There, a focus on comfort, avoiding expensive and futile care, and ensuring good communication among family members is integral to the palliative-care process. And while palliative care is commonly associated with the very end of life, advocates now consider palliation as a much longer-term treatment option, one that might provide guidance to care for patients who have a long-term terminal disease beginning at diagnosis. Better overall treatment for Ms. Watson that might have met her desires would have been palliation in the nursing home setting and a plan to avoid hospitalization, even in the face of acute diseases such as pneumonia, myocardial infarction (a heart attack), or exacerbation of a chronic disease such as heart failure.

Some of the biggest challenges to palliative care today are the strict standards imposed by Medicare for patients who elect to receive hospice care (which is one method of delivering palliative care). To qualify for Medicare-reimbursed hospice care, patients must be determined by their attending physician to have a life expectancy of less than six months; further, such patients must agree to forego any curative treatment options. It would be better to be more flexible on both counts. Physicians are notoriously inaccurate at predicting death in the short term; perhaps patients could self-designate as wanting palliative care while maintaining an option for receiving some types of acute-care management (for instance, treatment of a painful broken arm) while opting out of other types of acute-care management (for instance, treatment of pneumonia or myocardial infarction at the end of life). An example of current and future end-of-life care is shown in the graph on the following page (**Figure 11**).

While these changes are needed, enacting them requires legislative action. In the meantime the United States spends an inordinate amount of money on end-of-life care, patients who receive such care are often overtreated, and their family members are unhappy with the treatment. Longer-term hospice and palliative care would meet the needs and desires of patients and their families, unburden the acute-care delivery system, save patients and taxpayers money, and create a more efficient health-care system. As baby boomers transition to old age, this issue will become even more critical to address.

Figure 11. An example of current and future end-of-life care.

	Current	Future
Payment	For every test, visit, and hospitalization	For care management, including the development of advanced directives, and use of hospice or palliative care at the end of life
Face-to-face encounters are...	Revenue streams	Costs to the system
Hospice care...	Requires physician documentation that a patient is expected to die within 6 months	Could be entered when the patient determines, with physician advice, that patient is terminal
Hospice care...	Requires foregoing active treatment (including unrelated illness exacerbation)	Can include reasonable active treatment for exacerbations
The goal is...	To minimize care	To make the end of life more comfortable for the patient and family
Palliative care...	Occurs at the very end of life	Is more fluid and targets maintenance of comfort levels
Model looks like...	Patient has terminal illness → Physician finds that patient will die in < 6 months → Transfer to hospice care to minimize care → Acute exacerbations treated with palliation → Death	Patient has terminal illness → With physician guidance, patient chooses long-term palliation → Transfer to hospice care to maintain life quality → Acute exacerbations treated with desired treatment, informed by a shared decision-making process → Death

Chapter 12

Ideal-Care Vignette: An Industrial Revolution in Health-Care Delivery

Juanita Alvarez is a 67-year-old Hispanic female who lived in rural New Hampshire. She worked for 40 years in the hospitality industry prior to retiring at age 65; she lives on savings and social security, and she is enrolled in a Medicare Advantage program that includes coverage for eyeglasses, hearing aids, and medications. She obtained her health care through an integrated health care delivery system that is paid a fixed amount per year to provide for her health care needs, plus a bonus if the health of the population improves each year.

Juanita is generally pretty healthy, but she has two chronic conditions: diabetes and osteoarthritis. For both conditions, she is enrolled in registries so that the management and outcomes of these conditions can be monitored.

This morning, Juanita uses the integrated smartphone application to automatically input her finger-stick blood glucose reading. She waits a minute to get feedback from the application, which was also linked to her electronic medical record. Her glucose is a bit high, so the application recommends that she take two additional units of

113

regular insulin before having lunch. She does so and records the dose in the phone. By collecting data on her glucoses and insulin use over the past few years, the application was able to suggest day-to-day dosing changes that resulted in tight glucose control and a normal hemoglobin A1c level.

As she was inputting the insulin dose that she took, she received a text message from Pam, her health coach. Pam had received a notification that Juanita's blood glucose was a little high, so she sent Juanita a text asking her if she'd been able to exercise recently. Juanita responded that she had not been able to do so, but she was planning to go to the physical therapist that day. Pam wished her luck and reminded her about healthy eating habits and that it was import-ant that Juanita maintain tight control of her glucose because of the upcoming knee replacement surgery.

The pain from Juanita's knee osteoarthritis had become worse over the past three or four years. Her primary care physician had pre-scribed analgesics, and she had received some joint injections, but the pain was getting worse. Prior to being referred to surgery, Juan-ita had visited the shared decision-making center. There she first received information about the risks, benefits, and alternatives to knee replacement surgery. After considering the options and complet-ing a questionnaire that tested her decision quality, she decided to obtain the knee surgery. But then she went through a second process: the health care system showed her long-term outcomes and costs for patients with her characteristics associated with surgeries conducted in that health care system as well as three other local ones. When she looked at her anticipated out-of-pocket costs (which were based on 10 years of historical data) and her insurance coverage, she was a bit surprised to see that her out-of-pocket costs would have been higher had she chosen the hospital with the worst outcomes. "Why is that?" she asked the decision counselor.

"Insurance companies, who bear the financial brunt of costs asso-ciated with bad outcomes, have been allowed to design their benefits

packages to steer patients toward higher-quality, higher-value care. They're hoping that the higher costs, in concert with the worse outcomes, will persuade you to choose care in a system that provides higher-value care."

She chose the health care system where she got most of her care—the outcomes were excellent, and the out-of-pocket costs were minimal. She then met with the surgical team who reviewed her case, told her about the importance of keeping her diabetes in control (normal hemoglobin A1c levels in diabetic patients were associated with much better outcomes after knee replacement surgery), and gave her a day-by-day, hour-by-hour explanation of what she should expect during the brief hospital stay. She completed electronic overall health status and knee pain status. "Do you need information on my medical history or the medications that I take?" she asked.

"Not if they haven't changed recently," said Dr. Winters, the orthopedic surgeon. "We collect and update that information at each visit, to keep it accurate, but we only ask for the information we need, to minimize the burden on you."

Juanita also met with her physical therapist, who recommended exercises that she should begin before the surgery. "They make recovery much faster," the physical therapist said. There was a smartphone application that Juanita used to be reminded what exercises to do and when to do them. Juanita kept track of the exercise regimen and recorded it in the smartphone—that information was automatically integrated with her electronic medical record. As she had mentioned to Kim, her health coach, she'd not been doing as much of the exercises lately because of the increased pain.

When Juanita met with the physical therapist, she was given some guidance on how to minimize pain with the exercises. The physical therapist also indicated that she, along with a home health nurse, would be coming to Juanita's house daily for the first week after she was discharged from the hospital after her knee replacement. The physical therapist made sure Juanita had a walker and had practiced using it in the office before the surgery. Additionally, the physical therapist made sure Juanita had someone to help take care of her at home for a week or so. "My daughter will be staying with me," Juanita told her. "She's a great cook!"

Juanita's daughter drove her to the hospital on the day of surgery. She was the second case, scheduled for 9 a.m., and she went into the operating room at 9. By 1 p.m., she was in a room that contained a second bed so her daughter could sleep comfortably there. Juanita's hospital stay was uneventful. She was not awakened at night, as staff monitored her vital signs from a central pod. Rounds happened at 7:30 in the morning. "We used to do them at 5:30 or 6," Dr. Winters told her. "But patients were not getting adequate rest. It's important to recovery to get enough uninterrupted sleep."

Juanita left the hospital three days after surgery, following the anticipated course of hospitalization almost exactly as it had been explained to her. At home, she got home health nursing and physical therapy. A smartphone application monitored her pain and recommended when she take pain medications and how much to take, so as to minimize drowsiness and maximize effectiveness. Dr. Winters communicated with her via video each day—she was able to hold up the smartphone to show him the healing suture lines and to show him how much she was able to flex her knee.

Juanita's follow-up appointments at two, four, and six weeks were also done by phone. "Using your camera phone, we can examine you and check your wound. There's really no need for you to come in to see me," Dr. Winters said. "It's inconvenient for you and less efficient." Dr. Winters was able to show her how she was progressing and compare her progress to that of other patients with similar characteristics. She was right on track.

When Juanita received the hospital bill, it was only two pages long and was straightforward. The bill showed what they had anticipated she would have to pay out of pocket and what the actual out-of-pocket expenses were (they were about 5 percent less than had been anticipated). Because the hospital was reimbursed on a per-capita basis, with a fixed fee for special episodes of care such as knee replacement, there was simply a total charge for the episode that included the entire bundle of physical therapy and home health nursing. The slightly lower out-of-pocket costs were due to a somewhat more rapid recovery than had been anticipated; the home health nurse did not need to visit after four days because Juanita was doing so well and her daughter had been so effective at providing some of the care. The hospital shared the savings with Juanita by reducing her out-of-pocket costs.

Juanita completed online evaluations and satisfaction surveys using her smartphone. She found it was easier to respond to the questions if they were sent to her in small batches, every few hours. So that is what the survey program did. The data was fed into a national database that did not include any of Juanita's identifiable information but allowed researchers and health care systems to learn from the care provided and to help educate future patients like Juanita about the risks, benefits, and costs of care. Business intelligence and data analytics were used to anticipate any problems Juanita might experience following her surgery before she had any negative experiences.

Juanita and her daughter were delighted with the care they received, and after the surgery, Juanita's knee pain disappeared, allowing her to exercise more. Her smartphone application continued to monitor her insulin use and glucose levels, and because of the reduced pain and increased activity, she lost some weight and was able to change to oral management of her diabetes. She now feels the best she's felt in 20 years, and though she knows the health care system had a lot to do with her health improvement, she is particularly happy it provided the tools and treatments she needed, when she needed them, to help her maintain and improve her health.

Summary and Conclusions

We have written a book that used vignettes to capture common — but often unpleasant — experiences patients encounter in the current health care delivery process, provided a historical perspective designed to help patients make sense of those experiences, and outlined patient-centered care pathways that use new and exciting technological approaches to improve those experiences. We are mindful that what we propose will be threatening to the current medical industrial complex, but these changes are inevitable and are already occurring more rapidly than most appreciate. In fact, denying the change ignores the realities and only delays what a well-informed society wants and needs.

Key policy recommendations include aligning reimbursement to promote value creation in health care delivery, fostering transparency that allows patients to make informed decisions, promoting and rewarding informed-choice processes, and using behavioral-economics approaches and incentives to encourage patients to choose high-value health care.

Technological recommendations include using existing technology more effectively and efficiently, aligning and integrating diverse electronic medical records, and using the rapid evolution of new technologies to provide care when and where patients want the care provided and to improve the health care management of identified patient populations. A consumer-oriented health system—what a concept!

But patients need to be involved in—and indeed, drive—this industrial revolution in health care. We believe that besides supporting the policy and technology solutions we propose, patients can encourage the adoption of our recommendations by following the "What Do I Do?" patient checklist on the following pages. By stimulating health care insurers, providers, and delivery systems with this checklist, we believe these recommendations would be embedded into health care delivery processes more quickly. Health care value in the United States would improve, health care cost increases would become sustainable, and most importantly, patients would obtain more effective, more efficient, and more personal health care, when and where they want it, at costs they can afford.

The industrial revolution in health care has begun. Thanks for your help in accelerating this important revolution!

~Bill and Jim

THE "WHAT DO I DO?" CHECKLIST FOR PATIENTS

The checklist on the following page provides suggestions on what to ask and what to do if you are dissatisfied with the answers.

In making any health-care decision, we advocate considering the following facts:

1) Most health care illnesses are time limited and improve with the tincture of time; watchful waiting is an option.

2) Sometimes, when it comes to health care, less is more.

3) More health care spending is not associated with better health outcomes or patient satisfaction.

4) More health care spending is associated with worse health outcomes and less patient satisfaction.

5) One should request information (such as a test) only if one is prepared to use the results of that information. Having a test often leads to more invasive tests and/or procedures, which increases one's risk of more potential problems and/or complications.

The "What Do I Do?" Checklist

Situation	Ask
Deciding where to seek care	Does the health-care system or provider: • transparently and publicly display outcomes and costs for patients? • incorporate shared decision-making processes into the delivery process? • have the ability to show you how a decision might impact a patient like you? • have a patient portal so you can access your medical record?
Visiting a provider for the first time	Does the health-care system or provider: • have a process for collecting data so as to minimize your burden in completing forms? • have a process for monitoring and displaying changes in your health status and your outcomes over time? • provide multiple data-collection and communication formats so that your care can be monitored and you can access care when and how you want to?
Deciding whether to get a test	Can the health-care provider: • confirm that you are at risk for having the condition that the test is evaluating? • articulate how treatment will change if the test is positive or negative? • tell you the cost (both your out-of-pocket and that borne by your insurer) of the test?
Making a treatment decision	Does the health-care system or provider: • have a clear, shared, decision-making process that provides patients tools and measures their decision quality? • incorporate their own and regional outcomes and costs for patients into the shared decision-making processes? • have the ability to show you how a decision might impact a patient like you?
Staying in the hospital	Does the health-care system or provider: • demonstrate high-value care? • use longitudinal data to improve health-care outcomes? • communicate clearly and frequently? • provide good hotel-like services, including for accompanying family members? • minimize noise and interruptions?
Managing chronic disease or care at the end of life	Does the health-care system or provider: • transparently and publicly display outcomes and costs for patients? • incorporate shared decision-making processes into the delivery process? • incorporate their own and regional outcomes and costs for patients into the shared decision-making processes? • involve your family and friends, as you desire, in the care delivery and decision-making processes?
Understanding and interpreting the bill	Does the health-care system or provider: • provide an easily understandable and interpretable bill? • clearly state what you have paid and what you owe? • demonstrate cost savings that accrue to you by virtue of your choosing a high-value health-care delivery system or provider? • eradicate nonsensical, misleading discounts?

If the answer to any of these questions is 'no'…

1) Call your insurer, human resources benefits administrator, and the health care system or provider.

2) Ask "Why not?"

3) Suggest that they do so.

4) Suggest that the health care insurer fund such efforts (and that it will pay off!).

5) Suggest they read this book!

GLOSSARY OF TERMS

Affordable Care Act (ACA). Also known as "ObamaCare," the ACA broadened access to health insurance, beginning in 2014. This was achieved largely by developing insurance exchanges through which patients who were not covered by employee-sponsored health insurance could purchase their own insurance policy, the price of which was subsidized by the federal government. The ACA was designed to increase access to primary care providers and preventive care services, with the hope that this access would both reduce the need for acute-care services and reduce the prevalence of chronic diseases (by providing earlier intervention and prevention).

Benefits design. The way in which insurers craft the set of benefits that they offer. Health care benefits have several dimensions: what services are covered, where those services are covered (for instance, within a set network of hospitals or physicians, or perhaps anywhere), and how much the insured person has to pay for services they obtain (through copayments). Insurers can design the benefits packages they offer so as to direct patients toward high quality care, for instance by reducing copayment requirements when such providers are used for care. Further, insurers can disincentivize overuse of care—particularly futile or wasteful care—by increasing copayment requirements for those services.

Bundled payment. A bundled payment pays for a "bundle" of services, generally around an episode of care. For instance, a thirty-day bundled payment for a knee replacement surgery might include the preoperative assessment, the hospital stay, all physician costs, all follow-up visits within thirty days of discharge from the hospital, and treatment of any complications that might have occurred within the thirty-day window (including revisions that require rehospitalization). While bundled payments both limit risk for insurers and incentivize providers to be more efficient in care provision, there are some concerns that bundled payments could lower treatment thresholds (so that more patients who do not want or need the treatment end up getting it, causing utilization rates to rise) and exclude high-risk patients who warrant the intervention from getting it (because they are also at high risk for having a complication, which would cost the provider money, under a bundled payment agreement).

Capitation. Capitation is a reimbursement mechanism wherein a single payment, generally paid in advance, is the sole payment that is to cover all expenses generated in providing services for a particular patient, over a particular time period. Capitation incentives reduce utilization of health care services, as each service used is a cost under this form of reimbursement, as opposed to a revenue stream as when a fee-for-service reimbursement mechanism is used.

Coinsurance. Coinsurance is the amount that you, as an insured person, are required to pay that is sometimes a fixed amount and sometimes a percentage of a bill. For instance, Medicare Part B (which pays for physician visits) has a coinsurance rate of 20 percent; that means if the allowed reimbursement for a physician visit is one hundred dollars, you would be required to pay 20 percent — or twenty dollars — of that amount, and Medicare Part B would pay the rest. Sometimes coinsurance is applied per visit; for instance, many commercial insurance plans require that a patient pay a twenty-dollar copayment (which is coinsurance) for each outpatient visit.

Deductible. The deductible is the initial amount that you, as an insured person, are required to pay. Generally, the amount is a fixed amount for a specified service. For instance, in 2015, Medicare A (which pays for hospitalizations) had a $1,260 deductible for the first hospitalization that a Medicare beneficiary had that year. That means that whatever the cost of the hospitalization, the Medicare Part A beneficiary had to pay the first $1,260.

Diagnosis Related Group (DRG). A DRG is a reimbursement for a hospital stay. The DRG includes all nonphysician, hospital-related activities for the reason for admission; generally, this includes preoperative testing and the hospital stay. This form of reimbursement replaced a "cost-plus" form in 1981, wherein activities were itemized (such as nursing care for a day, meals consumed, and tests performed during the hospital stay) and were reimbursed individually. Such a system drove up both the costs of a hospitalization and the length of stay for a given hospitalization. By bundling all those costs, the DRG reimbursement mechanism incentivized shorter lengths of stay and less use of testing during hospitalization.

False-negative. A false-negative test is a test whose result is read as negative, although repeat tests indicate that the disease being tested for is present. In essence, false-negative tests incorrectly suggest — at least initially — that the patient does not have the disease or disorder that the test was ordered to identify. While tests are designed to minimize them, false-negatives happen sporadically. False-negative tests can provide a sense of complacency; unfortunately, the disease can progress while the patient believes he is disease free. An example is a negative colonoscopy test, when colon cancer is actually present.

False-positive. A false-positive test is a test whose result is read as positive, although repeat tests indicate that the disease being tested for is not present. In essence, false-positive tests incorrectly suggest—at least initially—that the patient has the disease or disorder that the test was ordered to identify. While tests are designed to minimize them, false-positives are much more likely when a person or population that is at very low risk for having the disease or disorder is tested. False-positive tests can cause considerable anxiety and discontent, as well as additional costs as the false-positive test is "worked up" with additional tests. An example is a false-positive hepatitis C test that requires follow-up and additional tests, but which the patient is ultimately determined not to have.

Fee-for-service. Fee-for-service is a reimbursement mechanism wherein each service is reimbursed separately. For instance, each time a physician sees a patient or orders a test, a new bill is generated and reimbursed. Such a reimbursement system incentivizes overuse of services.

Illness care. Illness care is care provided to treat active disease states, as opposed to care provided to prevent disease. Examples include operations, medications, emergency room visits, and urgent care visits.

Informed choice. Informed choice goes beyond shared decision-making by including additional information, particularly information on longitudinal outcomes of patients with similar characteristics who have—and have not—obtained the intervention being considered; information on the out-of-pocket costs of the different treatments; and outcomes and costs for different hospitals or health care systems in the area. In this way, informed choice not only helps patients make decisions about whether to pursue a particular treatment course, but also helps them decide where to obtain desired treatment.

Insurance premium. The insurance premium is the amount paid each month for insurance coverage. For most people in the United States, this is provided through employment, and the insurance premium is both split with your employer and deducted from your paycheck. With the ACA, the federal government subsidizes insurance premiums that are available through insurance exchanges for individuals and their families (the federal government also subsidizes insurance premiums provided by employers, as those premiums are considered employment costs and thereby reduce a company's tax burden).

Medicaid. A state-run and state- and federally funded health insurance program for people who have low incomes. The specific benefits of the program (what it will pay for) are determined by each state and therefore vary somewhat state to state. Eligibility, which is also determined by each state and therefore varies, is generally based on an individual's or family's income, as it relates to the federal poverty level (or some multiplier thereof).

Medicare. A federally funded health care insurance program for people who are eligible because they have contributed to Medicare through payroll taxation for forty quarters (ten years). People become eligible to have their health care funded (in part) by Medicare if they are determined to be disabled or if they have reached age sixty-five.

Preventive care. Preventive care is care provided to prevent disease, as opposed to care provided to treat disease. Examples include vaccinations, smoking-cessation services, and counseling on healthy lifestyles.

Rack rate. The rack rate is the amount charged for a particular treatment or visit. The reality is that virtually no one pays that amount. Rack rates are the basis from which significant discounts are provided to insurers and even individual payers who ask for the discounts. A rack rate can be easily conceptualized as the "original price" of an item of clothing at a discount outlet—the original price is relatively high, but the discounted price seems inexpensive, making consumers think they have saved a lot of money. In a similar fashion, health care organizations artificially inflate the "rack rate" prices so that they can offer substantial discounts to insurers and so that the insurers can claim they saved their insured population considerable sums of money.

Reimbursement. Reimbursement means the way that health care is paid. Different forms of reimbursement include fee-for-service, capitation, and bundled payments, descriptions of which are provided elsewhere in the glossary.

Shared decision-making. Shared decision-making is a process wherein risks and benefits of a particular treatment decision are shared with a patient (sometimes through written or videotaped materials) in order to enhance the patient's ability to make a treatment decision that is consistent with his goals and values. In essence, the process lays out the advantages and disadvantages of a particular treatment decision, evaluates the patient's values and priorities regarding the disease being treated, and tries to help reconcile those in the treatment decision. This process helps patients make decisions about whether to pursue a particular treatment course.

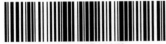

Made in the USA
Middletown, DE
24 February 2016